A Yoga Journal

A Yoga Journal

Lauren "Zehara" Haas, RYT

A Yoga Journal

Lauren "Zehara" Haas, RYT

Copyright Lauren Haas, 2013

Yoga pose illustrations by Charlotte Bradley, YogaFlavoredLife.com
from her 108 Yoga Poses collection.

ISBN-13: 978-1493774364

ISBN-10: 1493774360

Contents

Ideas: One year of monthly guided practices 9

Practice: Set intentions for your weekly practice 35

Classes: A year of after-class notes 89

Workshops & DVDs 143

Knowledge: Go deeper into yoga 157

    The 6 Systems of Yoga 158
    The 8 Limbs of Raja Yoga 159
    Yamas 160
    Niyamas 161
    Common yoga terms 162
    Sanskrit pose names 163
    Sun Salutation — *Surya Namaskar* 164
    Breathing Techniques 166
        Alternate Nostril Breath 166
        Breath of Joy 167
        Breath of Fire 168
    Chakras 170
    Koshas 172
    What is Ohm? 173
    About Meditation 174
    Guided Meditations 176
        Savasana (Relaxation) Meditation 177
        Energy Meditation 178
        Lovingkindness Meditation 180
        Koshas: A Falling Inward Meditation 181
        Dissipating Negative Emotions 182

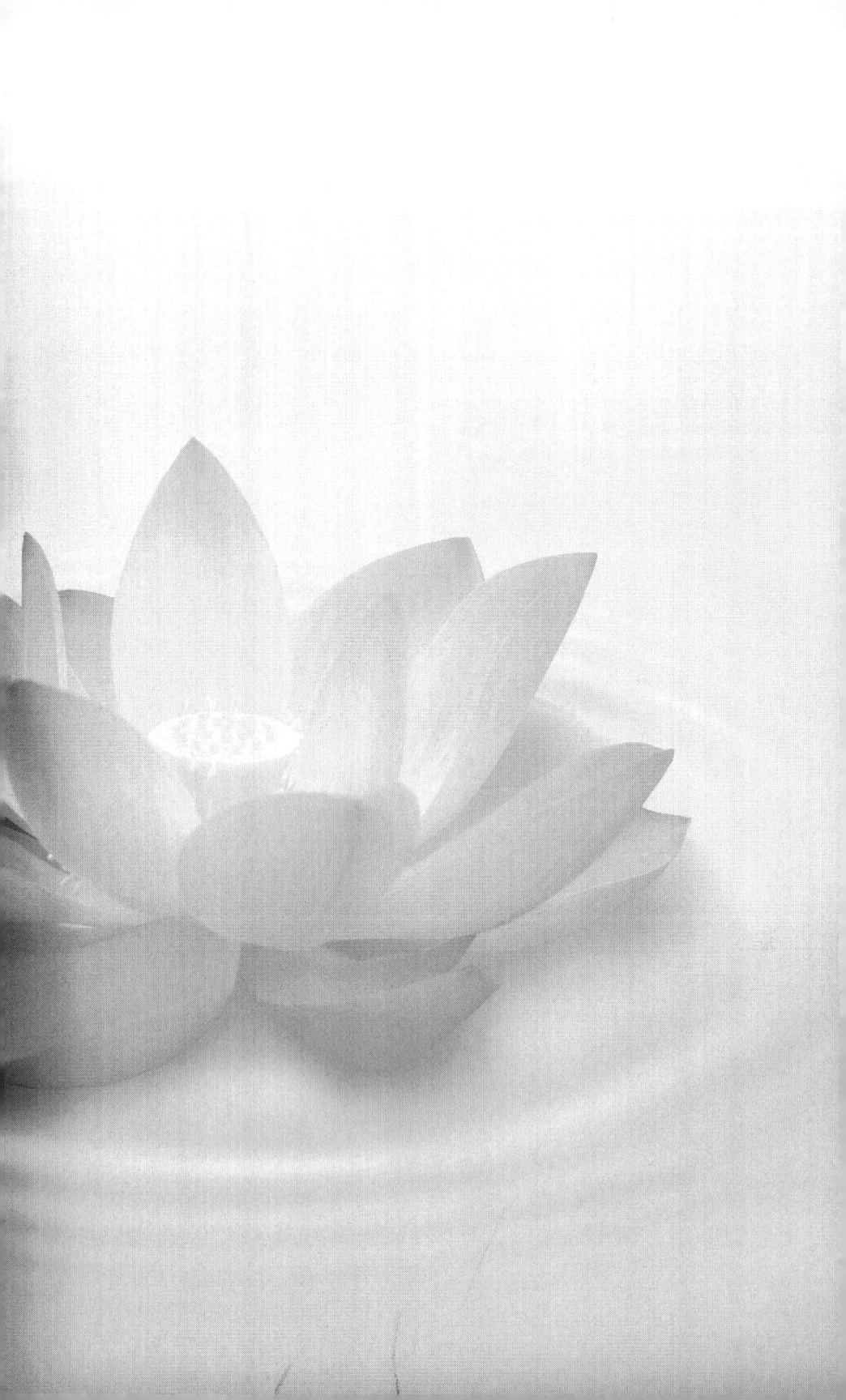

Acknowledgements

I'd like to thank my yoga teachers at Yandara Yoga Institute, including Craig Perkins and Christopher-Shane Perkins, for opening my body, mind and spirt fully to yoga.

Another of my certification teachers was Gay White, of The Yoga Garden in Berkely, who taught me alignment cues and partner work that were always present in my teaching.

I'd like to thank my mother, Mary Brent, with all my heart. She was my first and best yoga teacher. Thank you, Mom!

I found Charlotte Bradley's collection of 108 Yoga Pose Drawings at her website, YogaFlavoredLife.com, when I was a new teacher. I've used her stick figures to create notes for myself and handouts for my students for years. When I e-mailed Charlotte to ask about licensing the photos for use in this book, she was incredibly generous and encouraging.

To Beki Kellner-Walkup, thank you for patiently proofreading my manuscript and helping to catch the details that would have driven me nuts if they'd been missed.

Most importantly, I want to offer gratitude to all my students. Thank you for your loving patience at the times when you could have been critical. I learned so much from all of you.

Namasté,
Lauren

Ideas

One year of monthly guided practices & journaling

Bring curiosity and exploration to your mat
with these sequences.

If you aren't familiar with a suggested pose,
feel free to substitute a familiar one.

Trust yourself, and explore any ideas
that arise from within during your practice.

These sequences are meant to a supplement (not replace) live instruction.
A book cannot take the place of a teacher, and no attempts are made in these pages to give full
instructions for poses. You should learn new poses in person, from a qualified instructor.

Breathing the movement

Linking movement with breath is the heart of a yoga practice. Today, explore the way your breath dialogues with your movement.

Inhale as movements open your front body, and exhale when your ribcage and abdomen are being compressed.

Try doing Sun Salutations (see page 164 for a common version with breathing cues) or your favorite flow with your full focus on your breathing.

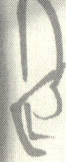

Stand in Mountain Pose with your eyes closed and palms together in front of your heart center. Feel the upward expansion within on each inhalation, and the downward pull of the exhalations.

Connect movement and breath by moving just your arms first. Let the inhalation lift your arms overhead. Feel how the in-breath opens your ribcage and enhances the sense of expansion. Exhale, bringing the arms down to your sides and returning them to prayer position, fully experiencing the downward pull of gravity as you exhale.

Practice Sun Salutations, or a flow, focusing fully on your breath. Allow each movement to be contained within a single breath. Initiate the breath before the movement, and complete the movement before completing the breath.

> In our uniquely human capacity to connect movement with breath and spiritual meaning, yoga is born.
> *-Gurmukh Kaur Khalsa*

A Yoga Journal

Write about your experience of connecting breath with movement. Were you able to quiet your mind more easily? Were you able to feel the flow of energy with your breath? What else did you experience?

Ideas

_____
_____
_____
_____
_____
_____
_____
_____
_____
_____
_____
_____
_____
_____
_____
_____

A Soothing Practice

Create a calming yoga practice for times when you feel agitated or anxious.

Begin standing and work your way down to the floor. Use music if you like.

Begin with standing poses to burn off energy, then balances to quiet the mind. Forward folds and child's pose settle the heart. Twists bring peace. End with alternate nostril breathing and legs up the wall pose. Aaaaah.

Begin with sun salutations, spending extra time in the forward folds and downward dogs.

Move through your favorite standing poses, like Warrior poses, Triangle, Side Angle Pose. Seek a balance between effort and surrender as you hold each pose for 3-5 breaths.

Challenge yourself with balance poses that suit your level. If balance poses are easy for you, work on transitioning between them. Try Tree Pose, Natarajasana, or Warrior 3.

Move to the floor and enjoy some seated twists and hip openers, like Pigeon. Breathe gently and do what feels good to you. Come into Child's Pose between other poses, breathing into your back body. Then sit for a few rounds of alternate nostril breathing (page 166).

Rest in Viparita Karani, , hips on a cushion or blanket and legs resting against the wall.

> Yoga is essentially a practice for your soul, working through the medium of your body.
> -Tara Fraser

How did your practice impact your emotions? What might you try differently next time?

_____
_____
_____
_____
_____
_____
_____
_____
_____
_____
_____
_____
_____
_____
_____
_____
_____
_____
_____
_____

An Energizing Practice

Whenever you're feeling lethargic or depressed, begin on the floor and build energy.

Start with music and a soothing supported child's pose that puts comforting pressure on the front of the body.

Use backbends to unlock energy from your heart center, and twists for balance. Finish with standing poses, an inversion or Sun Salutations and Breath of Joy.

Begin in child's pose, with a bolster or a couple of folded blankets or cushions under your chest and forehead. Just breathe and listen to music until you feel ready to move.

Move onto all fours for cat and cow poses to warm up the back body. Then take whatever gentle backbends suit your body, like locust, bridge, bow, or camel pose. Work up to more intense backbends like wheel if they are appropriate for your body.

Counter each backbend with a seated or reclining twist of your choice. Make each twist long and luxurious. Sprinkle a few forward bending poses in between, too, as it feels right to you.

Finish on a strong note. See if you can feel the triumphant energy of a Warrior pose, shoulderstand or Natarajasana, or savor a couple of leisurely sun salutations. Finish with Breath of Joy (page 167).

> *The yoga mat is a good place to turn when talk therapy and antidepressants aren't enough.*
> ~Amy Weintraub

Which poses bring you the most comfort when you feel down? Which poses energize you?

Get Grounded (Root Chakra)

Your root chakra is connected to safety, security, home. Relocating, fear of crime, and financial worries are situations that might disrupt the root chakra.

Root chakra upheaval can give you feelings of anxiety, panic, or indecisiveness.

Return to this practice any time you feel anxious or nervous and want to feel safe, grounded, calm and centered again.

If you know a flow or have a DVD that uses mostly standing poses, use it. Otherwise, use poses you're comfortable with (Mountain, Warrior 1, Warrior 2, Triangle), staying in each for 5 breaths.

Begin by centering in mountain pose. Feel your weight in all four corners of each foot. Adjust your hips until your weight feels even across your feet. Picture the imprint your feet are creating in your mat, deep and steady.

As you move through standing poses, keep bringing your awareness back to the feeling of your weight in your feet. Imagine roots growing through your legs and into the earth.

When you rest in savasana, connect with gravity on each exhalation. Feel your front body resting against your back body and your back body pressing against the floor.

> Warrior pose battles **inner weakness** and wins focus. You see that there is no war within you. You're on your own side, and you are your own strength.
> -*Terri Guillemets*

*See pages 170-171 for more information about the chakras.

A Yoga Journal

Write about your impressions of this grounding practice. Do you enjoy the feeling of connecting strongly with gravity?

_____
_____
_____
_____
_____
_____
_____
_____
_____
_____
_____
_____
_____
_____
_____
_____
_____

Ideas

Go With the Flow (Sacral Chakra)

The second chakra governs bodily fluids and opens us to receptivity, emotion, sensuality and pleasure.

Try hip openers and child's pose when you're dealing with emotional or sexual issues, or any time you need to find acceptance.

This slow, sleepy series heals the sacral chakra by easing your lower back, opening your hips, and encouraging you to surrender to gravity.

Begin in child's pose, with folded blankets under your torso and head. Surrender deeply to gravity. Focus on your lower back and hips moving in response to your breath. Stay until you feel tranquil.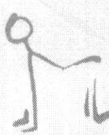

Enjoy some cat/cow stretches.

Press into downward dog, and raise one leg toward the ceiling. Feel the support from your lower belly. Bring that leg under your body for pigeon pose. Release to your elbows or to the floor and surrender, letting your hip soften deeply.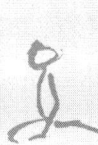

Repeat on the other side, moving slowly and fluidly between poses in any order you like, for as long as you wish.

Take child's pose with knees wide, easing into the strong resistance in your groin.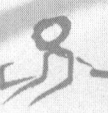

Add a seated straddle or your favorite hip openers.

End with a lengthy, supported child's pose, exactly as you began.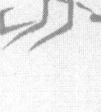

> Yoga is not about self-improvement, it's about self-acceptance.
>
> –Gurmukh Kaur Khalsa

*See pages 170-171 for more information about the chakras.

What role do you think your sacral chakra plays in your life? Does it feel too open, too constricted, or just right?

_____
_____
_____
_____
_____
_____
_____
_____
_____
_____
_____
_____
_____
_____
_____
_____
_____
_____
_____
_____

Ideas

Fiery Core (Navel Chakra)

Your navel chakra governs your metabolism and digestive system, as well as your self-esteem, will, and personal power.

A balanced third chakra is neither power-hungry or weak, neither fearful or angry. It is self-assured and at peace.

This sequence uses breath and core work to stimulate the navel chakra, then twists and backbends to relax and soften, for a balanced center.

> The harmonizing of opposing forces is a key aspect of yoga. Hot energy is united with cool energy, strong with soft, and masculine with feminine.
> ~Tara Fraser

Begin with Breath of Fire, described on page 168.

Come to Mountain pose. Warm up with a few Sun Salutations.

Spend 10-15 minutes practicing Boat Pose, Plank variations, or your favorite core-strengtheners. It's fine to use non-yoga core work as well, like crunches, leg lifts or sit ups, with yoga awareness. Try to keep your facial muscles relaxed and your breath steady and smooth.

Practice your favorite seated twists, and then reclining twists. Hold each pose for three to five breaths.

Lie down and come into Fish pose, cobra, or any light backbend you find comfortable to lengthen the abdominals. Hold for at least five slow breaths.

Relax a moment. Then take Bridge pose for five breaths.

Finish with reclining twists, then savasana.

*See pages 170-171 for more information about the chakras.

Does your navel chakra tends to be weak, or overactive? What kind of poses do you think will bring you balance?

Heart Openers (Heart Chakra)

A contracted heart chakra needs to learn to give and receive love. An overly-opened one is codependent, needing too much from others.

Learn to trust and open this chakra in supported backbends, where the heart is lifted higher than the head, and to reach out in active ones.

Forward bends help soothe a vulnerable heart chakra, especially when the front body is supported.

> Your task is not to
> seek for love,
> but merely to seek
> and find all the barriers
> within yourself
> that you have built.
> - Rumi

Begin with Breath of Joy (see page 167).

In Mountain Pose, bring your shoulders back and lengthen your neck. Imagine inhaling your heart center open and exhaling it closed.

Lie down with your lower shoulder blades elevated on a stack of folded blankets, shoulders and head on the floor. After several minutes, turn the blankets lengthwise to support your spine, from lower ribcage to head. In both poses, practice softening the heart center as you surrender.

Choose the active backbends that feel right for your body: Locust, Sphinx, Cobra, Upward-Facing Dog, Camel, Bridge, Fish, or Wheel. Periodically refresh your spine with a twist, then a forward bending pose.

Finally, rest in Child's Pose with folded blankets or cushions supporting your head and chest.

*See pages 170-171 for more information about the chakras.

Is your heart center closed and tight? Overly vulnerable? Many people move between the two extremes. How can you find balance, on or off the mat?

Transformation (Throat Chakra)

The throat chakra guides communication, including internal dialogue between the physical and spiritual planes.

Authentic personal expression is vital to the higher self. Music, dance, art, writing, and singing all encourage a healthy throat chakra.

On the mat, try neck and shoulder stretches, and connecting sound with movement. Experiment with chanting and singing.

Sit and become still. Then chant, sing or hum, as you prefer, bringing your awareness to the vibrations that fill you.

Allow the vibrations to fade away slowly. Practice your favorite gentle neck stretches.

Stand and step into Warrior 2. Inhale. As you exhale, chant a deep, vibrating Ohmmm sound and transition to Triangle pose.

Repeat several times on each side, feeling the release of energy during the exhalation.

Try Sun Salutation or your favorite flow series, chanting with each exhalation. If your practice includes shoulder stand and or plow, practice them after your flow.

Finish on the floor, holding a high bridge pose for 5-10 breaths. Rest briefly, then take Matsyasana for 5-10 breaths. Enjoy humming or chanting as you settle into Savasana.

> Yoga teaches us to cure
> what need not
> be endured
> and endure
> what cannot be cured.
> - B.K.S. Iyengar

*See pages 170-171 for more information about the chakras.

Do you have trouble expressing your true feelings? What were your emotional responses to making sounds during your practice?

Awakening (Third Eye & Crown Chakras)

Think of the third eye chakra, at the center of your forehead, as an eye that looks inward. This chakra rules dreams, imagination, intuition, and seeing beyond the physical realm.

Visualize the crown chakra, at the top of your skull, as a thousand-petaled lotus blossom. Or imagine your spirit connecting with the Divine as light and energy are allowed to pass thorough the crown.

After a slow, complete yoga practice, sit cross-legged and twist to your right, using your arms to support a tall, straight spine. Eyes closed, feel energy rising up from the base of your spine and forward to your forehead as you inhale, and feel the energy descend as you exhale. Repeat to the other side.

Sit cross-legged against a wall, with a block or cushion under your hips. Lick your finger and dampen the spot between and above your brows. Eyes closed, bring your awareness to that cool tingling spot. Focus again on your energy rising and falling with your breath.

When you feel focused, become aware of the crown of your head. Imagine feeling the tingle of energy there, and then draw that energy deep within as you inhale. As you exhale, imagine settling deeper into yourself. See if you can let go completely.

> Be a lamp to yourself.
> Be your own confidence.
> Hold on to the truth within yourself as to the only truth.
> - Buddha

*See pages 170-171 for more information about the chakras.

Are you generally open to things you cannot see? Do you feel ready to connect to your spirit, or to Divine energy?

A Yoga Journal

Balance

Balance starts decaying early. Yoga students are often surprised to find they've already lost the ability to stand on one foot!

Balance poses in yoga can help preserve or even restore this ability, preventing falls and injuries as we age.

Balance poses also teach focus (if your mind wanders, you will falter) as preparation for meditation, and serve as a metaphor for life skills.

> Life is a balance between
> what we can control
> and what we cannot.
> I am learning to live
> between effort
> and surrender.
> - Danielle Orner

Observe: Close your eyes and try to stand on one foot. Notice how much harder it is? *We use our vision to balance more than we know.*

Apply: Gaze at a stationary spot (drishti point) before you enter a balance pose, and keep your gaze steady. Don't move your head or eyes while balancing.

Observe: Close your eyes and stand on one foot again. Where do you feel muscles working to keep you balanced? *The muscles in your calves, ankles and feet are making tiny adjustments.*

Apply: Bring awareness to the soles of your feet. Learn which corner of the foot tries to lift, and press downward through that spot. Imagine the footprint you're creating in your mat. Keep it deep, steady, even.

When you wobble, your mind has wandered. Keep returning focus to the soles of your feet.

*See pages 170-171 for more information about the chakras.

Did your observations match the ones given? Does gazing at a drishti point and focusing your awareness in your feet help you with balance poses? Does balancing frighten you?

_____
_____
_____
_____
_____
_____
_____
_____
_____
_____
_____
_____
_____
_____
_____
_____
_____

Gentle Hip Openers

Yoga teaches us that our bodies, minds and spirits are connected.

Opening the hips not only prevents injuries in the knees and lower back, but helps release emotion and memory that are trapped deep in the fascia and muscles.

If your hips are tight, practice being gentle and patient with your body. Don't move into pain. Take time to surrender to gravity in each pose.

> Now feel the space in your joints...Open yourself up to everything you sense and feel... Feel ...the energy that is your true nature.
> -Eckhart Tolle

Lie on your back and place the ball of your right foot into a strap. Stretch that foot to the ceiling. Don't pull on the strap. Use strap to give your foot something to press against as you actively lengthen your leg.

Turn your leg at the hip so your toes point left (pigeon-toed) and move both ends of the strap to your left hand. Keeping both hips on the floor, take the straight right leg across your body to the left until you feel resistance. Hold for 30 seconds.

Transfer the strap ends to your right hand and open the leg out to the right as far as you can, using a block or bolster for support. Hold 30 seconds or more.

Release the leg and lie flat. Observe the sensation of one leg feeling longer than the other.

Repeat on the other side. Enjoy your other favorite hip openers, and finish with pigeon pose.

A Yoga Journal

Describe how opening your hips affects your emotional state. When would be the best times for you to practice hip openers?

Ideas

Meditation for Beginners

Most people believe that they are made of body, mind, and spirit. We know our bodies, and our minds. But have you met your spirit?

Meditation quiets your body and your mind so you can turn your focus inward and see what else is present.

When you've learned to let go of tension in the body, bring that practice to the mind. Be present and let go. Over and over again.

> Yoga is the cessation of the movements of the mind. Then there is abiding in the Seer's own form.
> *-Patanjali, The Yoga Sutras of Patanjali*

Comfort is critical, so if traditional seated poses don't work for you, elevate your hips on a cushion and support your back against a wall, or use a chair. Your spine should be straight, your head upright.

Focus on your body. Feel your clothing against your skin. Behind closed eyelids, lower your gaze and let your awareness drop from your brain into your heart center.

With each exhalation, let your awareness sink deeper inside yourself. Keep letting go. As thoughts arise, brush them aside, returning to your breath.

Look inward as if you are looking into a dark room and waiting for your eyes to adjust to the darkness, as if you will see something wonderful soon.

Stay patient and curious. Enjoy the process and the refreshing mental openness.

See more meditation advice beginning on page 174

When thoughts intrude, are they mostly about the past or the future? Is it hard to be patient with yourself? What else would you like to note about this experience?

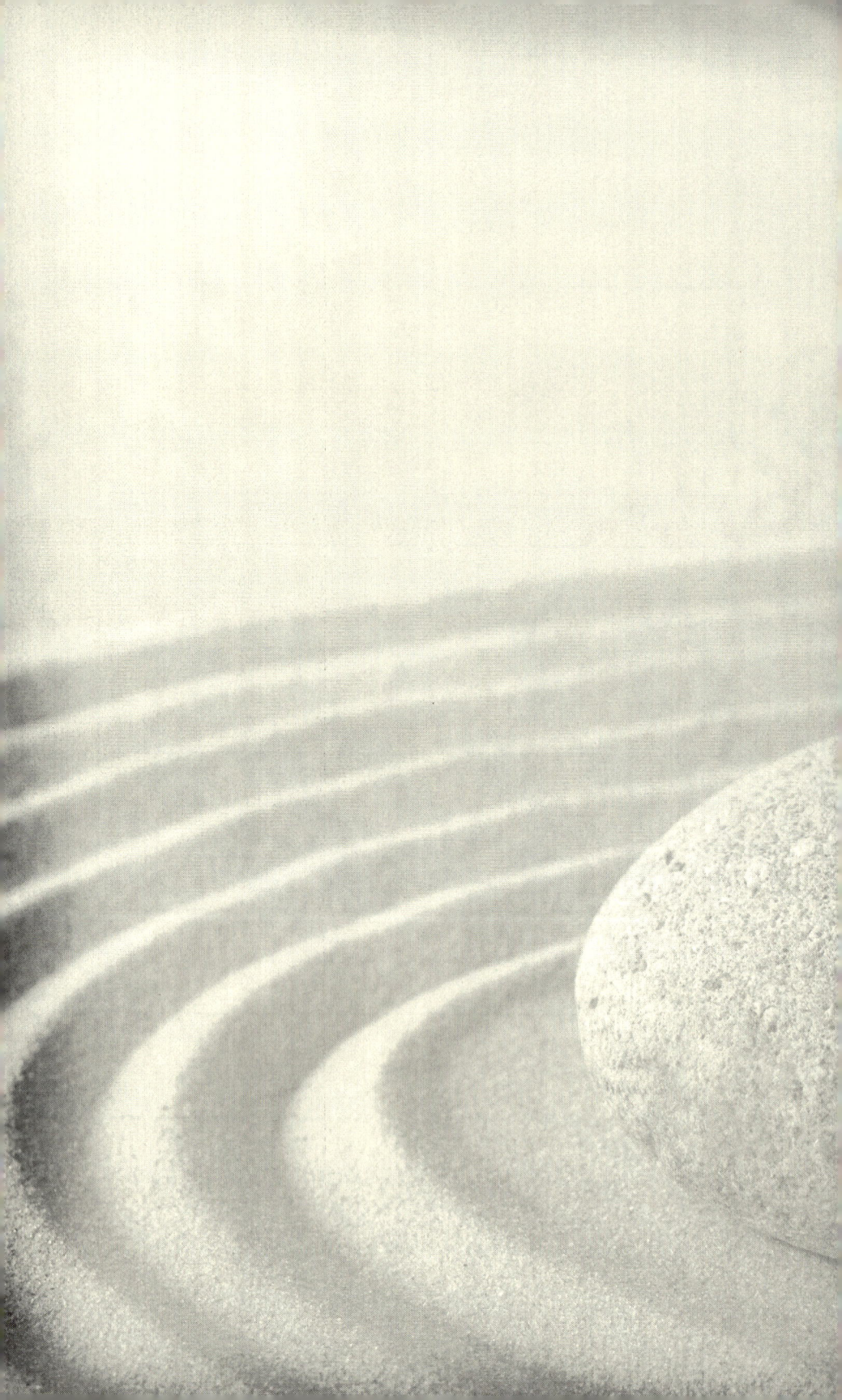

A Yoga Journal

Practice

Set intentions for your weekly practice and journal your growth

A Yoga Journal

Week of **Jan 1st 2021**

This week's practice

Before: My Intentions

Focus: __breath and Posture__

Music: _____

How long to practice daily: __15 - 30 mins.__

Things to remember: __dont push yourself - ease in at first__

After: My Thoughts

How much did I challenge myself? (circle)   1 2 3 4 5 6 7 8 9 10

Intention vs. practice _____

How it felt: _____

Next week: _____

A Yoga Journal

Week of _____

This week's practice

Before: My Intentions

Focus: _____

Music: _____

How long to practice daily: _____

Things to remember: _____
_____
_____

After: My Thoughts

How much did I challenge myself? (circle) 1 2 3 4 5 6 7 8 9 10

Intention vs. practice _____
_____

How it felt: _____
_____
_____
_____
_____
_____

Next week: _____
_____

A Yoga Journal

Week of _____

This week's practice

Before: My Intentions

Focus: _____

Music: _____

How long to practice daily: _____

Things to remember: _____

_____

_____

After: My Thoughts

How much did I challenge myself? (circle)   1 2 3 4 5 6 7 8 9 10

Intention vs. practice _____

_____

How it felt: _____

_____

_____

_____

_____

_____

Next week: _____

_____

A Yoga Journal

Week of _____

This week's practice

Before: My Intentions

Focus: _____

Music: _____

How long to practice daily: _____

Things to remember: _____
_____
_____

After: My Thoughts

How much did I challenge myself? (circle) 1 2 3 4 5 6 7 8 9 10

Intention vs. practice _____
_____

How it felt: _____
_____
_____
_____
_____
_____

Next week: _____
_____

Practice

A Yoga Journal

Week of _____

This week's practice

Before: My Intentions

Focus: _____

Music: _____

How long to practice daily: _____

Things to remember: _____

_____

_____

After: My Thoughts

How much did I challenge myself? (circle) 1 2 3 4 5 6 7 8 9 10

Intention vs. practice _____

_____

How it felt: _____

_____

_____

_____

_____

Next week: _____

_____

A Yoga Journal   41

Week of _____

This week's practice

Before: My Intentions

Focus: _____

Music: _____

How long to practice daily: _____

Things to remember: _____

_____

_____

After: My Thoughts

How much did I challenge myself? (circle) 1 2 3 4 5 6 7 8 9 10

Intention vs. practice _____

_____

How it felt: _____

_____

_____

_____

_____

_____

Next week: _____

_____

Practice

A Yoga Journal

Week of _____

This week's practice

Before: My Intentions

Focus: _____

Music: _____

How long to practice daily: _____

Things to remember: _____
_____
_____

After: My Thoughts

How much did I challenge myself? (circle) 1 2 3 4 5 6 7 8 9 10

Intention vs. practice _____
_____

How it felt: _____
_____
_____
_____
_____
_____

Next week: _____
_____

A Yoga Journal

Week of _____

This week's practice

Before: My Intentions

Focus: _____

Music: _____

How long to practice daily: _____

Things to remember: _____
_____
_____

After: My Thoughts

How much did I challenge myself? (circle) 1 2 3 4 5 6 7 8 9 10

Intention vs. practice _____
_____

How it felt: _____
_____
_____
_____
_____
_____

Next week: _____
_____

Practice

A Yoga Journal

Week of _____

This week's practice

Before: My Intentions

Focus: _____

Music: _____

How long to practice daily: _____

Things to remember: _____
_____
_____

After: My Thoughts

How much did I challenge myself? (circle)   1 2 3 4 5 6 7 8 9 10

Intention vs. practice _____
_____

How it felt: _____
_____
_____
_____
_____
_____
_____

Next week: _____
_____

A Yoga Journal

Week of _____

This week's practice

Before: My Intentions

Focus: _____

Music: _____

How long to practice daily: _____

Things to remember: _____
_____
_____

Practice

After: My Thoughts

How much did I challenge myself? (circle) 1 2 3 4 5 6 7 8 9 10

Intention vs. practice _____
_____

How it felt: _____
_____
_____
_____
_____
_____

Next week: _____
_____

A Yoga Journal

Week of _____

This week's practice

Before: My Intentions

Focus: _____

Music: _____

How long to practice daily: _____

Things to remember: _____
_____
_____

After: My Thoughts

How much did I challenge myself? (circle) 1 2 3 4 5 6 7 8 9 10

Intention vs. practice _____
_____

How it felt: _____
_____
_____
_____
_____
_____

Next week: _____
_____

A Yoga Journal   47

Week of _____

This week's practice

Before: My Intentions

Focus: _____

Music: _____

How long to practice daily: _____

Things to remember: _____
_____
_____

After: My Thoughts

How much did I challenge myself? (circle)   1 2 3 4 5 6 7 8 9 10

Intention vs. practice _____
_____

How it felt: _____
_____
_____
_____
_____
_____

Next week: _____
_____

Practice

A Yoga Journal

Week of _____

This week's practice

Before: My Intentions

Focus: _____

Music: _____

How long to practice daily: _____

Things to remember: _____
_____
_____

After: My Thoughts

How much did I challenge myself? (circle)   1 2 3 4 5 6 7 8 9 10

Intention vs. practice _____
_____

How it felt: _____
_____
_____
_____
_____
_____

Next week: _____
_____

A Yoga Journal

Week of _____

This week's practice

Before: My Intentions

Focus: _____

Music: _____

How long to practice daily: _____

Things to remember: _____

_____

_____

After: My Thoughts

How much did I challenge myself? (circle) 1 2 3 4 5 6 7 8 9 10

Intention vs. practice _____

_____

How it felt: _____

_____

_____

_____

_____

_____

Next week: _____

_____

Practice

A Yoga Journal

Week of _____

This week's practice

Before: My Intentions

Focus: _____

Music: _____

How long to practice daily: _____

Things to remember: _____
_____
_____

After: My Thoughts

How much did I challenge myself? (circle) 1 2 3 4 5 6 7 8 9 10

Intention vs. practice _____
_____

How it felt: _____
_____
_____
_____
_____
_____

Next week: _____
_____

A Yoga Journal

Week of _____

This week's practice

Before: My Intentions

Focus: _____

Music: _____

How long to practice daily: _____

Things to remember: _____

_____

_____

After: My Thoughts

How much did I challenge myself? (circle)   1 2 3 4 5 6 7 8 9 10

Intention vs. practice _____

_____

How it felt: _____

_____

_____

_____

_____

Next week: _____

_____

Practice

A Yoga Journal

Week of _____

This week's practice

Before: My Intentions

Focus: _____

Music: _____

How long to practice daily: _____

Things to remember: _____

_____

_____

After: My Thoughts

How much did I challenge myself? (circle) 1 2 3 4 5 6 7 8 9 10

Intention vs. practice _____

_____

How it felt: _____

_____

_____

_____

_____

_____

Next week: _____

_____

A Yoga Journal

Week of _____

This week's practice

Before: My Intentions

Focus: _____

Music: _____

How long to practice daily: _____

Things to remember: _____
_____
_____

After: My Thoughts

How much did I challenge myself? (circle) 1 2 3 4 5 6 7 8 9 10

Intention vs. practice _____
_____

How it felt: _____
_____
_____
_____
_____
_____
_____

Next week: _____
_____

A Yoga Journal

Week of _____

This week's practice

Before: My Intentions

Focus: _____

Music: _____

How long to practice daily: _____

Things to remember: _____
_____
_____

After: My Thoughts

How much did I challenge myself? (circle) 1 2 3 4 5 6 7 8 9 10

Intention vs. practice _____
_____

How it felt: _____
_____
_____
_____
_____
_____

Next week: _____
_____

A Yoga Journal

Week of _____

This week's practice

Before: My Intentions

Focus: _____

Music: _____

How long to practice daily: _____

Things to remember: _____
_____
_____

After: My Thoughts

How much did I challenge myself? (circle) 1 2 3 4 5 6 7 8 9 10

Intention vs. practice _____
_____

How it felt: _____
_____
_____
_____
_____

Next week: _____
_____

Practice

A Yoga Journal

Week of _____

This week's practice

Before: My Intentions

Focus: _____

Music: _____

How long to practice daily: _____

Things to remember: _____
_____
_____

After: My Thoughts

How much did I challenge myself? (circle)   1 2 3 4 5 6 7 8 9 10

Intention vs. practice _____
_____

How it felt: _____
_____
_____
_____
_____
_____
_____

Next week: _____
_____

A Yoga Journal

Week of _____

This week's practice

Before: My Intentions

Focus: _____

Music: _____

How long to practice daily: _____

Things to remember: _____
_____
_____

After: My Thoughts

How much did I challenge myself? (circle) 1 2 3 4 5 6 7 8 9 10

Intention vs. practice _____
_____

How it felt: _____
_____
_____
_____
_____
_____

Next week: _____
_____

A Yoga Journal

Week of _____

This week's practice

Before: My Intentions

Focus: _____

Music: _____

How long to practice daily: _____

Things to remember: _____
_____
_____

After: My Thoughts

How much did I challenge myself? (circle) 1 2 3 4 5 6 7 8 9 10

Intention vs. practice _____
_____

How it felt: _____
_____
_____
_____
_____
_____

Next week: _____
_____

A Yoga Journal

Week of _____

This week's practice

Before: My Intentions

Focus: _____

Music: _____

How long to practice daily: _____

Things to remember: _____
_____
_____

After: My Thoughts

How much did I challenge myself? (circle) 1 2 3 4 5 6 7 8 9 10

Intention vs. practice _____
_____

How it felt: _____
_____
_____
_____
_____
_____

Next week: _____
_____

Practice

A Yoga Journal

Week of _____

This week's practice

Before: My Intentions

Focus: _____

Music: _____

How long to practice daily: _____

Things to remember: _____
_____
_____

After: My Thoughts

How much did I challenge myself? (circle)   1 2 3 4 5 6 7 8 9 10

Intention vs. practice _____
_____

How it felt: _____
_____
_____
_____
_____
_____

Next week: _____
_____

A Yoga Journal

Week of _____

This week's practice

Before: My Intentions

Focus: _____

Music: _____

How long to practice daily: _____

Things to remember: _____

_____

_____

After: My Thoughts

How much did I challenge myself? (circle) 1 2 3 4 5 6 7 8 9 10

Intention vs. practice _____

_____

How it felt: _____

_____

_____

_____

_____

_____

Next week: _____

_____

Practice

A Yoga Journal

Week of _____

This week's practice

Before: My Intentions

Focus: _____

Music: _____

How long to practice daily: _____

Things to remember: _____
_____
_____

After: My Thoughts

How much did I challenge myself? (circle)   1 2 3 4 5 6 7 8 9 10

Intention vs. practice _____
_____

How it felt: _____
_____
_____
_____
_____
_____

Next week: _____
_____

A Yoga Journal   63

Week of _____

This week's practice

Before: My Intentions

Focus: _____

Music: _____

How long to practice daily: _____

Things to remember: _____
_____
_____

After: My Thoughts

How much did I challenge myself? (circle) 1 2 3 4 5 6 7 8 9 10

Intention vs. practice _____
_____

How it felt: _____
_____
_____
_____
_____
_____

Next week: _____
_____

Practice

A Yoga Journal

Week of _____

This week's practice

Before: My Intentions

Focus: _____

Music: _____

How long to practice daily: _____

Things to remember: _____

_____

_____

After: My Thoughts

How much did I challenge myself? (circle) 1 2 3 4 5 6 7 8 9 10

Intention vs. practice _____

_____

How it felt: _____

_____

_____

_____

_____

_____

Next week: _____

_____

A Yoga Journal

Week of _____

This week's practice

Before: My Intentions

Focus: _____

Music: _____

How long to practice daily: _____

Things to remember: _____

_____

_____

After: My Thoughts

How much did I challenge myself? (circle)   1 2 3 4 5 6 7 8 9 10

Intention vs. practice _____

_____

How it felt: _____

_____

_____

_____

_____

_____

Next week: _____

_____

Practice

A Yoga Journal

Week of _____

This week's practice

Before: My Intentions

Focus: _____

Music: _____

How long to practice daily: _____

Things to remember: _____
_____
_____

After: My Thoughts

How much did I challenge myself? (circle)   1 2 3 4 5 6 7 8 9 10

Intention vs. practice _____
_____

How it felt: _____
_____
_____
_____
_____
_____

Next week: _____
_____

A Yoga Journal

Week of _____

This week's practice

Before: My Intentions

Focus: _____

Music: _____

How long to practice daily: _____

Things to remember: _____

_____

_____

After: My Thoughts

How much did I challenge myself? (circle)   1 2 3 4 5 6 7 8 9 10

Intention vs. practice _____

_____

How it felt: _____

_____

_____

_____

_____

_____

Next week: _____

_____

A Yoga Journal

Week of _____

This week's practice

Before: My Intentions

Focus: _____

Music: _____

How long to practice daily: _____

Things to remember: _____
_____
_____

After: My Thoughts

How much did I challenge myself? (circle)   1 2 3 4 5 6 7 8 9 10

Intention vs. practice _____
_____

How it felt: _____
_____
_____
_____
_____
_____

Next week: _____
_____

A Yoga Journal

Week of _____

This week's practice

Before: My Intentions

Focus: _____

Music: _____

How long to practice daily: _____

Things to remember: _____
_____
_____

After: My Thoughts

How much did I challenge myself? (circle)   1 2 3 4 5 6 7 8 9 10

Intention vs. practice _____
_____

How it felt: _____
_____
_____
_____
_____
_____

Next week: _____
_____

Practice

A Yoga Journal

Week of _____

This week's practice

Before: My Intentions

Focus: _____

Music: _____

How long to practice daily: _____

Things to remember: _____

_____

_____

After: My Thoughts

How much did I challenge myself? (circle) 1 2 3 4 5 6 7 8 9 10

Intention vs. practice _____

_____

How it felt: _____

_____

_____

_____

_____

_____

Next week: _____

_____

A Yoga Journal

Week of _____

This week's practice

Before: My Intentions

Focus: _____

Music: _____

How long to practice daily: _____

Things to remember: _____
_____
_____

After: My Thoughts

How much did I challenge myself? (circle) 1 2 3 4 5 6 7 8 9 10

Intention vs. practice _____
_____

How it felt: _____
_____
_____
_____
_____
_____

Next week: _____
_____

Practice

A Yoga Journal

Week of _____

This week's practice

Before: My Intentions

Focus: _____

Music: _____

How long to practice daily: _____

Things to remember: _____

_____

_____

After: My Thoughts

How much did I challenge myself? (circle) 1 2 3 4 5 6 7 8 9 10

Intention vs. practice _____

_____

How it felt: _____

_____

_____

_____

_____

Next week: _____

_____

A Yoga Journal

Week of _____

This week's practice

Before: My Intentions

Focus: _____

Music: _____

How long to practice daily: _____

Things to remember: _____

_____

_____

After: My Thoughts

How much did I challenge myself? (circle)   1 2 3 4 5 6 7 8 9 10

Intention vs. practice _____

_____

How it felt: _____

_____

_____

_____

_____

_____

Next week: _____

_____

Practice

A Yoga Journal

Week of _____

This week's practice

Before: My Intentions

Focus: _____

Music: _____

How long to practice daily: _____

Things to remember: _____
_____
_____

After: My Thoughts

How much did I challenge myself? (circle)   1 2 3 4 5 6 7 8 9 10

Intention vs. practice _____
_____

How it felt: _____
_____
_____
_____
_____
_____

Next week: _____
_____

A Yoga Journal

Week of _____

This week's practice

Before: My Intentions

Focus: _____

Music: _____

How long to practice daily: _____

Things to remember: _____

_____

_____

After: My Thoughts

How much did I challenge myself? (circle)   1 2 3 4 5 6 7 8 9 10

Intention vs. practice _____

_____

How it felt: _____

_____

_____

_____

_____

_____

Next week: _____

_____

Practice

A Yoga Journal

Week of _____

This week's practice

Before: My Intentions

Focus: _____

Music: _____

How long to practice daily: _____

Things to remember: _____
_____
_____

After: My Thoughts

How much did I challenge myself? (circle) 1 2 3 4 5 6 7 8 9 10

Intention vs. practice _____
_____

How it felt: _____
_____
_____
_____
_____
_____

Next week: _____
_____

A Yoga Journal   77

Week of _____

This week's practice

Before: My Intentions

Focus: _____

Music: _____

How long to practice daily: _____

Things to remember: _____
_____
_____

After: My Thoughts

How much did I challenge myself? (circle)   1 2 3 4 5 6 7 8 9 10

Intention vs. practice _____
_____
_____

How it felt: _____
_____
_____
_____
_____
_____
_____

Next week: _____
_____

Practice

A Yoga Journal

Week of _____

This week's practice

Before: My Intentions

Focus: _____

Music: _____

How long to practice daily: _____

Things to remember: _____
_____
_____

After: My Thoughts

How much did I challenge myself? (circle) 1 2 3 4 5 6 7 8 9 10

Intention vs. practice _____
_____

How it felt: _____
_____
_____
_____
_____

Next week: _____
_____

A Yoga Journal

Week of _____

This week's practice

Before: My Intentions

Focus: _____

Music: _____

How long to practice daily: _____

Things to remember: _____

_____

_____

After: My Thoughts

How much did I challenge myself? (circle) 1 2 3 4 5 6 7 8 9 10

Intention vs. practice _____

_____

How it felt: _____

_____

_____

_____

_____

_____

Next week: _____

_____

A Yoga Journal

Week of _____

This week's practice

Before: My Intentions

Focus: _____

Music: _____

How long to practice daily: _____

Things to remember: _____
_____
_____

After: My Thoughts

How much did I challenge myself? (circle)   1 2 3 4 5 6 7 8 9 10

Intention vs. practice _____
_____

How it felt: _____
_____
_____
_____
_____
_____

Next week: _____
_____

A Yoga Journal

Week of _____

This week's practice

Before: My Intentions

Focus: _____

Music: _____

How long to practice daily: _____

Things to remember: _____

_____

_____

After: My Thoughts

How much did I challenge myself? (circle) 1 2 3 4 5 6 7 8 9 10

Intention vs. practice _____

_____

How it felt: _____

_____

_____

_____

_____

_____

Next week: _____

_____

Practice

A Yoga Journal

Week of _____

This week's practice

Before: My Intentions

Focus: _____

Music: _____

How long to practice daily: _____

Things to remember: _____
_____
_____

After: My Thoughts

How much did I challenge myself? (circle)   1 2 3 4 5 6 7 8 9 10

Intention vs. practice _____
_____

How it felt: _____
_____
_____
_____
_____
_____

Next week: _____
_____

A Yoga Journal

Week of _____

This week's practice

Before: My Intentions

Focus: _____

Music: _____

How long to practice daily: _____

Things to remember: _____

_____

After: My Thoughts

How much did I challenge myself? (circle) 1 2 3 4 5 6 7 8 9 10

Intention vs. practice _____

_____

How it felt: _____

_____

_____

_____

_____

_____

Next week: _____

_____

Practice

A Yoga Journal

Week of _____

This week's practice

Before: My Intentions

Focus: _____

Music: _____

How long to practice daily: _____

Things to remember: _____
_____
_____

After: My Thoughts

How much did I challenge myself? (circle)   1 2 3 4 5 6 7 8 9 10

Intention vs. practice _____
_____

How it felt: _____
_____
_____
_____
_____
_____

Next week: _____
_____

A Yoga Journal

Week of _____

This week's practice

Before: My Intentions

Focus: _____

Music: _____

How long to practice daily: _____

Things to remember: _____
_____
_____

After: My Thoughts

How much did I challenge myself? (circle)   1 2 3 4 5 6 7 8 9 10

Intention vs. practice _____
_____

How it felt: _____
_____
_____
_____
_____
_____

Next week: _____
_____

Practice

A Yoga Journal

Week of _____

This week's practice

Before: My Intentions

Focus: _____

Music: _____

How long to practice daily: _____

Things to remember: _____
_____
_____

After: My Thoughts

How much did I challenge myself? (circle)   1 2 3 4 5 6 7 8 9 10

Intention vs. practice _____
_____

How it felt: _____
_____
_____
_____
_____
_____

Next week: _____
_____

A Yoga Journal

Week of _____

This week's practice

Before: My Intentions

Focus: _____

Music: _____

How long to practice daily: _____

Things to remember: _____

_____

_____

After: My Thoughts

How much did I challenge myself? (circle)   1 2 3 4 5 6 7 8 9 10

Intention vs. practice _____

_____

How it felt: _____

_____

_____

_____

_____

_____

Next week: _____

_____

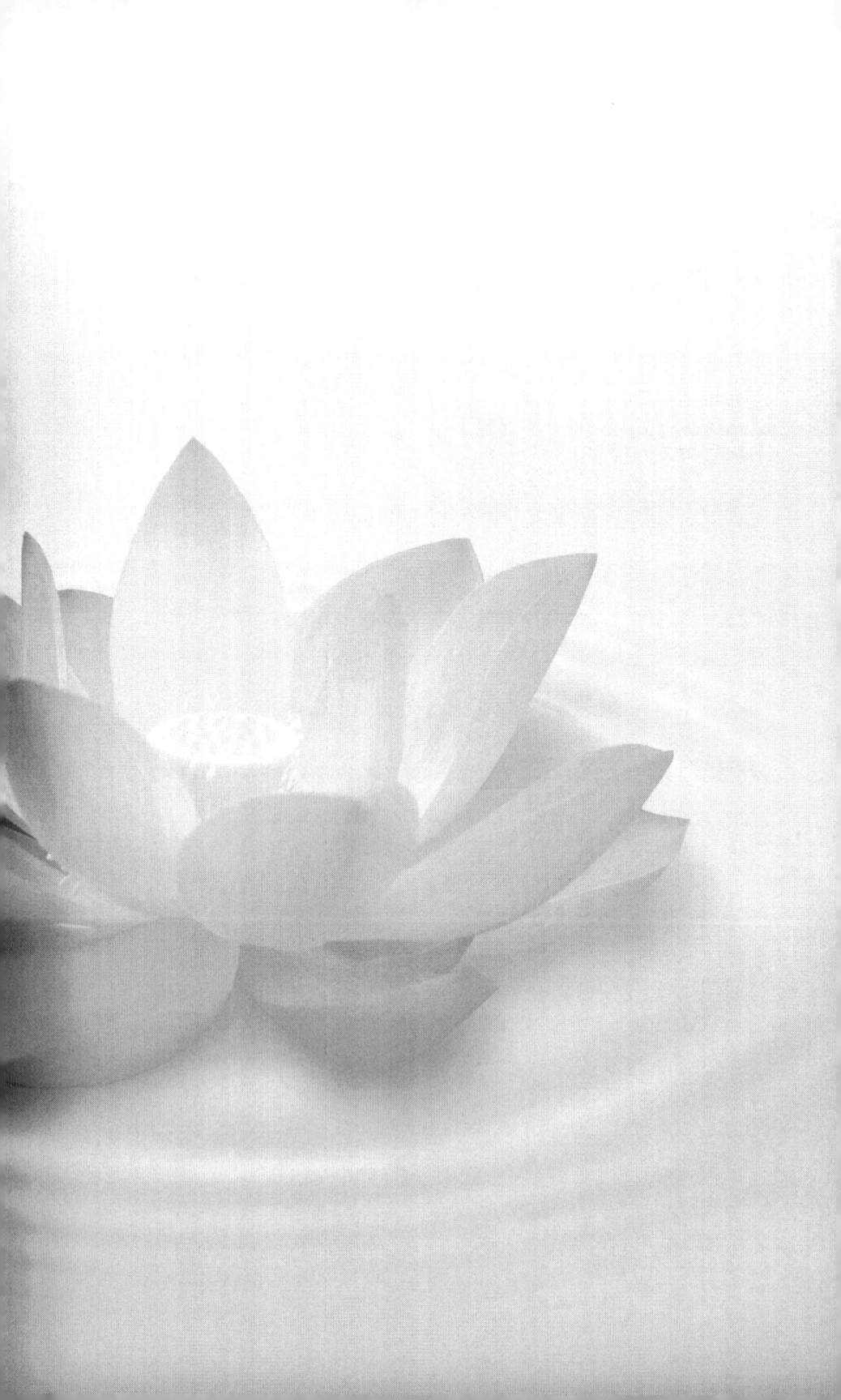

Classes

A year of after-class notes.
Witness your progress and remember
all you've encountered in class.

Date _____

Class Notes

Music I loved today: _____

How I felt on the way into class: _____

How I felt on the way out of class: _____

Most difficult new skill: _____

Skill that's getting easier: _____

Add to home practice: _____

Notes: _____

A Yoga Journal

Date _____

Class Notes

Music I loved today: _____

How I felt on the way into class: _____

How I felt on the way out of class: _____

Most difficult new skill: _____

Skill that's getting easier: _____

Add to home practice: _____

Notes: _____
_____
_____
_____
_____
_____
_____
_____
_____
_____
_____

Classes

Date _____

Class Notes

Music I loved today: _____

How I felt on the way into class: _____

How I felt on the way out of class: _____

Most difficult new skill: _____

Skill that's getting easier: _____

Add to home practice: _____

Notes: _____
_____
_____
_____
_____
_____
_____
_____
_____
_____
_____

A Yoga Journal

Date _____

Class Notes

Music I loved today: _____

How I felt on the way into class: _____

How I felt on the way out of class: _____

Most difficult new skill: _____

Skill that's getting easier: _____

Add to home practice: _____

Notes: _____

_____

_____

_____

_____

_____

_____

_____

_____

_____

_____

_____

Classes

Date _____

Class Notes

Music I loved today: _____

How I felt on the way into class: _____

How I felt on the way out of class: _____

Most difficult new skill: _____

Skill that's getting easier: _____

Add to home practice: _____

Notes: _____
_____
_____
_____
_____
_____
_____
_____
_____
_____
_____
_____
_____
_____

Date _____

Class Notes

Music I loved today: _____

How I felt on the way into class: _____

How I felt on the way out of class: _____

Most difficult new skill: _____

Skill that's getting easier: _____

Add to home practice: _____

Notes: _____

Date _____

Class Notes

Music I loved today: _____

How I felt on the way into class: _____

How I felt on the way out of class: _____

Most difficult new skill: _____

Skill that's getting easier: _____

Add to home practice: _____

Notes: _____
_____
_____
_____
_____
_____
_____
_____
_____
_____
_____
_____
_____

Date _____

Class Notes

Music I loved today: _____

How I felt on the way into class: _____

How I felt on the way out of class: _____

Most difficult new skill: _____

Skill that's getting easier: _____

Add to home practice: _____

Notes: _____
_____
_____
_____
_____
_____
_____
_____
_____
_____
_____
_____

Date _____

Class Notes

Music I loved today: _____

How I felt on the way into class: _____

How I felt on the way out of class: _____

Most difficult new skill: _____

Skill that's getting easier: _____

Add to home practice: _____

Notes: _____

_____

_____

_____

_____

_____

_____

_____

_____

_____

_____

Date _____

Class Notes

Music I loved today: _____

How I felt on the way into class: _____

How I felt on the way out of class: _____

Most difficult new skill: _____

Skill that's getting easier: _____

Add to home practice: _____

Notes: _____
_____
_____
_____
_____
_____
_____
_____
_____
_____
_____
_____
_____

Date _____

Class Notes

Music I loved today: _____

How I felt on the way into class: _____

How I felt on the way out of class: _____

Most difficult new skill: _____

Skill that's getting easier: _____

Add to home practice: _____

Notes: _____
_____
_____
_____
_____
_____
_____
_____
_____
_____
_____
_____

Date _____

Class Notes

Music I loved today: _____

How I felt on the way into class: _____

How I felt on the way out of class: _____

Most difficult new skill: _____

Skill that's getting easier: _____

Add to home practice: _____

Notes: _____

_____

_____

_____

_____

_____

_____

_____

_____

_____

_____

_____

_____

A Yoga Journal

Date _____

Class Notes

Music I loved today: _____

How I felt on the way into class: _____

How I felt on the way out of class: _____

Most difficult new skill: _____

Skill that's getting easier: _____

Add to home practice: _____

Notes: _____

_____

_____

_____

_____

_____

_____

_____

_____

_____

_____

_____

Date _____

Class Notes

Music I loved today: _____

How I felt on the way into class: _____

How I felt on the way out of class: _____

Most difficult new skill: _____

Skill that's getting easier: _____

Add to home practice: _____

Notes: _____

Classes

Date _____

Class Notes

Music I loved today: _____

How I felt on the way into class: _____

How I felt on the way out of class: _____

Most difficult new skill: _____

Skill that's getting easier: _____

Add to home practice: _____

Notes: _____

Date _____

Class Notes

Music I loved today: _____

How I felt on the way into class: _____

How I felt on the way out of class: _____

Most difficult new skill: _____

Skill that's getting easier: _____

Add to home practice: _____

Notes: _____
_____
_____
_____
_____
_____
_____
_____
_____
_____
_____
_____
_____

Classes

Date _____

Class Notes

Music I loved today: _____

How I felt on the way into class: _____

How I felt on the way out of class: _____

Most difficult new skill: _____

Skill that's getting easier: _____

Add to home practice: _____

Notes: _____
_____
_____
_____
_____
_____
_____
_____
_____
_____
_____
_____
_____
_____

Date _____

Class Notes

Music I loved today: _____

How I felt on the way into class: _____

How I felt on the way out of class: _____

Most difficult new skill: _____

Skill that's getting easier: _____

Add to home practice: _____

Notes: _____
_____
_____
_____
_____
_____
_____
_____
_____
_____
_____

Date _____

Class Notes

Music I loved today: _____

How I felt on the way into class: _____

How I felt on the way out of class: _____

Most difficult new skill: _____

Skill that's getting easier: _____

Add to home practice: _____

Notes: _____
_____
_____
_____
_____
_____
_____
_____
_____
_____
_____
_____
_____
_____

Date _____

Class Notes

Music I loved today: _____

How I felt on the way into class: _____

How I felt on the way out of class: _____

Most difficult new skill: _____

Skill that's getting easier: _____

Add to home practice: _____

Notes: _____
_____
_____
_____
_____
_____
_____
_____
_____
_____
_____
_____

Date _____

Class Notes

Music I loved today: _____

How I felt on the way into class: _____

How I felt on the way out of class: _____

Most difficult new skill: _____

Skill that's getting easier: _____

Add to home practice: _____

Notes: _____
_____
_____
_____
_____
_____
_____
_____
_____
_____
_____
_____
_____

Date _____

Class Notes

Music I loved today: _____

How I felt on the way into class: _____

How I felt on the way out of class: _____

Most difficult new skill: _____

Skill that's getting easier: _____

Add to home practice: _____

Notes: _____

Date _____

Class Notes

Music I loved today: _____

How I felt on the way into class: _____

How I felt on the way out of class: _____

Most difficult new skill: _____

Skill that's getting easier: _____

Add to home practice: _____

Notes: _____

_____

_____

_____

_____

_____

_____

_____

_____

_____

_____

_____

_____

Class Notes

Date _____

Music I loved today: _____

How I felt on the way into class: _____

How I felt on the way out of class: _____

Most difficult new skill: _____

Skill that's getting easier: _____

Add to home practice: _____

Notes: _____
_____
_____
_____
_____
_____
_____
_____
_____
_____
_____
_____

Date _____

Class Notes

Music I loved today: _____

How I felt on the way into class: _____

How I felt on the way out of class: _____

Most difficult new skill: _____

Skill that's getting easier: _____

Add to home practice: _____

Notes: _____

Date _____

Class Notes

Music I loved today: _____

How I felt on the way into class: _____

How I felt on the way out of class: _____

Most difficult new skill: _____

Skill that's getting easier: _____

Add to home practice: _____

Notes: _____

_____

_____

_____

_____

_____

_____

_____

_____

_____

_____

_____

Date _____

Class Notes

Music I loved today: _____

How I felt on the way into class: _____

How I felt on the way out of class: _____

Most difficult new skill: _____

Skill that's getting easier: _____

Add to home practice: _____

Notes: _____

_____
_____
_____
_____
_____
_____
_____
_____
_____
_____
_____

Date _____

Class Notes

Music I loved today: _____

How I felt on the way into class: _____

How I felt on the way out of class: _____

Most difficult new skill: _____

Skill that's getting easier: _____

Add to home practice: _____

Notes: _____
_____
_____
_____
_____
_____
_____
_____
_____
_____
_____
_____
_____

Classes

Date _____

Class Notes

Music I loved today: _____

How I felt on the way into class: _____

How I felt on the way out of class: _____

Most difficult new skill: _____

Skill that's getting easier: _____

Add to home practice: _____

Notes: _____

_____

_____

_____

_____

_____

_____

_____

_____

_____

_____

_____

Date _____

Class Notes

Music I loved today: _____

How I felt on the way into class: _____

How I felt on the way out of class: _____

Most difficult new skill: _____

Skill that's getting easier: _____

Add to home practice: _____

Notes: _____
_____
_____
_____
_____
_____
_____
_____
_____
_____
_____
_____

Date _____

Class Notes

Music I loved today: _____

How I felt on the way into class: _____

How I felt on the way out of class: _____

Most difficult new skill: _____

Skill that's getting easier: _____

Add to home practice: _____

Notes: _____

A Yoga Journal

Date _____

Class Notes

Music I loved today: _____

How I felt on the way into class: _____

How I felt on the way out of class: _____

Most difficult new skill: _____

Skill that's getting easier: _____

Add to home practice: _____

Notes: _____
_____
_____
_____
_____
_____
_____
_____
_____
_____
_____

A Yoga Journal

Date _____

Class Notes

Music I loved today: _____

How I felt on the way into class: _____

How I felt on the way out of class: _____

Most difficult new skill: _____

Skill that's getting easier: _____

Add to home practice: _____

Notes: _____
_____
_____
_____
_____
_____
_____
_____
_____
_____
_____
_____
_____
_____

Date _____

Class Notes

Music I loved today: _____

How I felt on the way into class: _____

How I felt on the way out of class: _____

Most difficult new skill: _____

Skill that's getting easier: _____

Add to home practice: _____

Notes: _____
_____
_____
_____
_____
_____
_____
_____
_____
_____
_____
_____
_____

Date _____

Class Notes

Music I loved today: _____

How I felt on the way into class: _____

How I felt on the way out of class: _____

Most difficult new skill: _____

Skill that's getting easier: _____

Add to home practice: _____

Notes: _____

Date _____

Class Notes

Music I loved today: _____

How I felt on the way into class: _____

How I felt on the way out of class: _____

Most difficult new skill: _____

Skill that's getting easier: _____

Add to home practice: _____

Notes: _____
_____
_____
_____
_____
_____
_____
_____
_____
_____
_____
_____

Date _____

Class Notes

Music I loved today: _____

How I felt on the way into class: _____

How I felt on the way out of class: _____

Most difficult new skill: _____

Skill that's getting easier: _____

Add to home practice: _____

Notes: _____

_____

_____

_____

_____

_____

_____

_____

_____

_____

_____

_____

Date _____

Class Notes

Music I loved today: _____

How I felt on the way into class: _____

How I felt on the way out of class: _____

Most difficult new skill: _____

Skill that's getting easier: _____

Add to home practice: _____

Notes: _____
_____
_____
_____
_____
_____
_____
_____
_____
_____

Classes

Date _____

Class Notes

Music I loved today: _____

How I felt on the way into class: _____

How I felt on the way out of class: _____

Most difficult new skill: _____

Skill that's getting easier: _____

Add to home practice: _____

Notes: _____

A Yoga Journal

Date _____

Class Notes

Music I loved today: _____

How I felt on the way into class: _____

How I felt on the way out of class: _____

Most difficult new skill: _____

Skill that's getting easier: _____

Add to home practice: _____

Notes: _____
_____
_____
_____
_____
_____
_____
_____
_____
_____
_____
_____

Date _____

Class Notes

Music I loved today: _____

How I felt on the way into class: _____

How I felt on the way out of class: _____

Most difficult new skill: _____

Skill that's getting easier: _____

Add to home practice: _____

Notes: _____
_____
_____
_____
_____
_____
_____
_____
_____
_____
_____
_____

Date _____

Class Notes

Music I loved today: _____

How I felt on the way into class: _____

How I felt on the way out of class: _____

Most difficult new skill: _____

Skill that's getting easier: _____

Add to home practice: _____

Notes: _____
_____
_____
_____
_____
_____
_____
_____
_____
_____
_____

Classes

Date _____

Class Notes

Music I loved today: _____

How I felt on the way into class: _____

How I felt on the way out of class: _____

Most difficult new skill: _____

Skill that's getting easier: _____

Add to home practice: _____

Notes: _____
_____
_____
_____
_____
_____
_____
_____
_____
_____
_____

Date _____

Class Notes

Music I loved today: _____

How I felt on the way into class: _____

How I felt on the way out of class: _____

Most difficult new skill: _____

Skill that's getting easier: _____

Add to home practice: _____

Notes: _____
_____
_____
_____
_____
_____
_____
_____
_____
_____
_____

Date _____

Class Notes

Music I loved today: _____

How I felt on the way into class: _____

How I felt on the way out of class: _____

Most difficult new skill: _____

Skill that's getting easier: _____

Add to home practice: _____

Notes: _____
_____
_____
_____
_____
_____
_____
_____
_____
_____
_____
_____

Date _____
Class Notes

Music I loved today: _____

How I felt on the way into class: _____

How I felt on the way out of class: _____

Most difficult new skill: _____

Skill that's getting easier: _____

Add to home practice: _____

Notes: _____

_____

_____

_____

_____

_____

_____

_____

_____

_____

_____

Date _____

Class Notes

Music I loved today: _____

How I felt on the way into class: _____

How I felt on the way out of class: _____

Most difficult new skill: _____

Skill that's getting easier: _____

Add to home practice: _____

Notes: _____
_____
_____
_____
_____
_____
_____
_____
_____
_____
_____
_____
_____

Date _____

Class Notes

Music I loved today: _____

How I felt on the way into class: _____

How I felt on the way out of class: _____

Most difficult new skill: _____

Skill that's getting easier: _____

Add to home practice: _____

Notes: _____
_____
_____
_____
_____
_____
_____
_____
_____
_____
_____
_____

Date _____

Class Notes

Music I loved today: _____

How I felt on the way into class: _____

How I felt on the way out of class: _____

Most difficult new skill: _____

Skill that's getting easier: _____

Add to home practice: _____

Notes: _____
_____
_____
_____
_____
_____
_____
_____
_____
_____
_____
_____

Date _____

Class Notes

Music I loved today: _____

How I felt on the way into class: _____

How I felt on the way out of class: _____

Most difficult new skill: _____

Skill that's getting easier: _____

Add to home practice: _____

Notes: _____
_____
_____
_____
_____
_____
_____
_____
_____
_____
_____

Date _____

Class Notes

Music I loved today: _____

How I felt on the way into class: _____

How I felt on the way out of class: _____

Most difficult new skill: _____

Skill that's getting easier: _____

Add to home practice: _____

Notes: _____

Date _____

Class Notes

Music I loved today: _____

How I felt on the way into class: _____

How I felt on the way out of class: _____

Most difficult new skill: _____

Skill that's getting easier: _____

Add to home practice: _____

Notes: _____

A Yoga Journal

Workshops & DVDs

Record notes, practice reminders, and people you meet at a dozen workshops (or DVDs)

Workshops & DVDs

Special Topic

A Yoga Journal

Date: _____

Instructor: _____

Topic: _____

Light Bulb Moments:
_____
_____
_____

To Practice:
_____
_____
_____
_____
_____
_____
_____
_____
_____
_____
_____

Notes

A Yoga Journal

People

Name — Facebook/e-mail/phone

the instructor

Workshops & DVDs

Special Topic

A Yoga Journal

Date: _____

Instructor: _____

Topic: _____

Light Bulb Moments:
_____
_____
_____

To Practice:
_____
_____
_____
_____
_____
_____
_____
_____
_____
_____

A Yoga Journal

Notes

People

Name Facebook/e-mail/phone

the instructor

Workshops & DVDs

A Yoga Journal

Special Topic

Date: _____

Instructor: _____

Topic: _____

Light Bulb Moments:
_____
_____
_____

To Practice:
_____
_____
_____
_____
_____
_____
_____
_____
_____
_____
_____
_____

Notes

A Yoga Journal

People

Name — Facebook/e-mail/phone

the instructor

Workshops & DVDs

Special Topic

A Yoga Journal

Date: _____

Instructor: _____

Topic: _____

Light Bulb Moments:

_____
_____
_____

To Practice:

_____
_____
_____
_____
_____
_____
_____
_____
_____
_____
_____

Notes

A Yoga Journal

People

Name — Facebook/e-mail/phone

the instructor

Workshops & DVDs

Special Topic

Date: _____

Instructor: _____

Topic: _____

Light Bulb Moments:

_____
_____
_____

To Practice:

_____
_____
_____
_____
_____
_____
_____
_____
_____
_____
_____

Notes

A Yoga Journal

People

Name — Facebook/e-mail/phone

the instructor

Workshops & DVDs

Special Topic

A Yoga Journal

Date: _____

Instructor: _____

Topic: _____

Light Bulb Moments:
_____
_____
_____

To Practice:
_____
_____
_____
_____
_____
_____
_____
_____
_____
_____
_____
_____

Notes

A Yoga Journal

People

Name — Facebook/e-mail/phone

the instructor

Workshops & DVDs

A Yoga Journal 157

Knowledge
Go deeper into yoga with readings and meditations.

Information

The 6 Systems of Yoga

The word 'yoga' means 'to yoke' or join together. The intention of yoga is to join the mind, body, and spirit.

Yoga is NOT a religion. Yoga does not dictate a set of religious beliefs or worship a deity. Yoga can be practiced within any religion, or apart from any religious beliefs at all. Some people use yoga to feel closer to God and to their spirit. Other people just do yoga poses for exercise and relaxation. *Your intention defines your relationship to yoga.*

There are six systems of Yoga, different ways to practice and work toward enlightenment and union with spirit.

- **Hatha Yoga** (ha=Sun, tha=Moon) prepares the mind for enlightenment through the path of the body. It includes asana (postures), breath control, and other physical practices. This encompasses most yoga classes taught in the United States.

- **Raja Yoga** (Royal Yoga) encompasses 8 limbs, including asana, for those who want to go deeper in their yoga practice. We'll talk about the limbs in more detail on the next page.

- **Bhakti Yoga** (Yoga of the heart, of devotion) seeks enlightenment through feelings of unconditional love, compassion, humility, and the intention to merge with the Divine.

- **Jnana Yoga** (Yoga of Knowledge) strives for enlightenment through the path of the mind, study, and self-inquiry.

- **Kriya Yoga** (Yoga of action). *Kriyas* are specific movements, mantras and meditations designed to remove obstructions.

- **Karma yoga** (Yoga of service). Karma yoga consists of acts of service, a selfless desire to help others.

The 8 Limbs of Raja Yoga

Many people enjoy yoga as a purely physical practice of stretching, strengthening and finding peace within the body. The physical postures of yoga are a complete practice for them.

But yoga postures represent just one of the eight limbs of Raja Yoga, as it was defined by Patanjali in his *Yoga Sutra* around 200 AD. Patanjali described an eight-step process for settling the restlessness of the mind and finding lasting peace.

- **Yama**: Universal morality (see page 160)
- **Niyama**: Personal observances (see page 161)
- **Asana**: Body postures
- **Pranayama**: Breathing exercises (see page 166)
- **Pratyahara**: Control of the senses
- **Dharana**: Concentration and cultivating inner awareness (see pages 176 for meditations to build Pratyahara and Dharma)
- **Dhyana**: Devotion, meditation on the Divine
- **Samadhi**: Union with the Divine

Patanjali considered these limbs of yoga to be an *Eightfold Path to Enlightenment*, and intended for anyone seeking enlightenment to work on all eight limbs, starting with observing the Yamas and Niyamas to purify his spirit and working toward incorporating all eight limbs.

Most Westerners are familiar with the third limb, the physical practice of yoga (Hatha Yoga). Most schools and styles of yoga practiced in the US are forms of Hatha Yoga. There is often more difference between individual teachers within the same style than between the schools.

For a more thorough discussion of all eight of Patanjali's limbs, I recommend B.K.S. Iyengar's book, *Light on Yoga*.

Yamas

The five Yamas are about ethics and morality, how you conduct yourself on a daily basis.

Ahimsa: Nonviolence

Ahimsa means treating ourselves and others with gentleness. Learn to recognize negativity that might cause you to inflict harm carelessly. We practice *Ahimsa* on the mat when we are gentle with ourselves, don't move into pain; and avoid harmful self-talk during our practice.

Satya: Truthfulness

Honesty in our communication with others is essential — when it is not harmful or unkind. Absolute honesty with oneself is often far more difficult than honesty with others. We practice *Satya* on the mat when we are honest about the limits of our strength, flexibility and patience.

Asteya: Nonstealing

Asteya means not taking that which is not freely given or earned. Besides the obvious — don't steal — it means not demanding people's time or attention beyond what is freely given. Avoid taking more than your fair share in relationships, from the planet, from society.

Brahmacharya: Continence

This yama was traditionally interpreted to mean sexual abstinence, reserving sexual energy for spiritual pursuits. Today it is often interpreted more loosely as sexual restraint, responsible sexual behavior.

Aparigraha: Non-hoarding, Non-grasping

Take only what is necessary, don't accumulate possessions. Trust yourself and/or God to provide what you will need in the future. Do not collect more wealth or objects than you need right now.

Niyamas

The Niyamas are spiritual observances, daily practices that strive toward spiritual purity and remembrance. The Niyamas are a set of rules that guide us toward our spirit.

Saucha: Purity, Cleanliness

Saucha means keeping the internal and external body clean (the body is the temple of the spirit). It also implies purity of thought, cleansing the mind of jealousy, hatred, passion, anger, lust, greed, delusion and pride.

Samtosa: Contentment

Cultivating contentment means learning to focus on the positive in life and accept the negative. *Samtosa* teaches us to practice gratitude, enjoy little things, and resist the urge to feed the negative energy within ourselves.

Tapas: Spiritual Discipline

Tapas literally means 'to burn' and implies a fiery commitment of energy to spiritual goals. *Tapas* is the energy you bring to working every day on your mat or your meditation cushion, the discipline you bring to your diet or to the daily practice of these Yamas and Niyamas.

Svadhyaya: Self-Study and Study of Scriptures

Looking inward, finding the remnants of selfishness, ego, jealousy, and negativity within oneself is essential if you are to burn those energies away. Studying spiritual texts, or religious scriptures of your choice, also leads to insight.

Isvara Pranidhana: Surrender to your Higher Power

No matter how you choose to define your higher power, at some point you must learn to let go of attachment to the outcome of your actions. Do your best, be your best, but know the results are out of your hands.

Common yoga terms

Agni: Fire. Usually refers to the cleansing digestive fire, or metabolism, which assimilates food and burns off waste and toxins. Can be visualized as a pilot light behind the navel.

Asana: Seat. Yoga position or pose, also called *yogasana*.

Bandha: Muscles are contracted to create energy lock in a specific area and move energy upward. Most common are *Mula Bandha* (at the perineum/cervix), *Uddiyana Bandha* (at the diaphragm), and *Jalandhara Bandha* (at the throat).

Chakra: Wheel-shaped energy centers along the core of the body. Points where mind, body and spirit intersect. (see page 170)

Dharma: Traveling one's right path through life; duty.

Guru: Spiritually enlightened soul, a teacher, who can enlighten others.

Hatha yoga: The physical practice of yoga, using body postures to align body mind and spirit.

Kundalini: Potential energy and inherent consciousness.

Nadi: Energy channels in the body, similar to the meridians in acupuncture

Om or Ohm or Aum: The universal mantra; cosmic vibration of the universe; (see page 173)

Prana: Energy force sustaining life in the body, similar to Chi in acupuncture.

Pranayama: Breath control techniques intended to regulate energy flow within the body (see page 166)

Samskara: Impressions stored in the mind that form the basis of our beliefs, attitudes and personality. Habitual patterns of thought.

Savasana: Relaxation pose, at the end of a yoga class or practice. *Savasana* allows time to internalize yoga experiences.

Yoga: State of union between two opposites — body and mind; individual and universal consciousness; a process of uniting the body and mind to achieve supreme awareness and enlightenment

Vinyasa: A series of poses with fluid transitions. A yoga flow.

Sanskrit pose names

Yogis use Sanskrit names for poses for the same reason botanists use Latin names for plants — clarity. Common names sometimes vary by region, or even by teacher. In this book, I've used common names where I think they are universally understood. Occasionally I've used the Sanskrit name for clarity.

Standing Poses
Tadasana: Mountain Pose
Uttanasana: Forward Fold Pose
Virabhadrasana I: Warrior One Pose
Virabhadrasana 2: Warrior Two Pose
Utthita Trikonasana: Extended Triangle Pose
Utthita Parsvakonasana: Extended Side Angle Pose
Vriksasana: Tree Pose
Utkatasana: Chair Pose or Powerful Pose
Adho Mukha Svanasana: Downward Facing Dog Pose

On the Mat
Baddha Konasana: Bound Angle Pose
Dandasana: Staff Pose
Bhujangasana: Cobra Pose
Sukhasana: Easy Pose (Seated cross-legged)
Setu Bandha Sarvangasana: Bridge Pose
Eka Pada Rajakapotasana: One-legged King Pigeon Pose
Urdhva Dhanurasana: Wheel Pose (classic backbend)
Balasana: Child's Pose

Inversions
Salamba Sarvangasana: Supported Shoulderstand
Salamba Sirsasana: Supported Headstand
Adho Mukha Vrksasana: Handstand

Relaxation
Viparita Karani: Legs-up-the-wall pose
Savasana: Relaxation Pose, Corpse Pose

Sun Salutation —Surya Namaskar

The *Salute to the Sun* is the most common *vinyasa*, or moving sequence of poses, and is often used to warm up the body at the beginning of a yoga class or practice. Repetitions of Sun Salutation can also be a complete practice, followed by savasana, resting pose. There are many variations, but here is a common version.

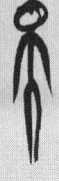

Tadasana
Exhale in the pose

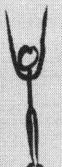

Inhale, stretching arms up
Utthita Tadasana

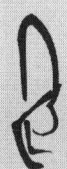

Exhale, folding at hips into
Uttanasana (Forward Fold)
Inhale, lifting halfway up with back flat, then

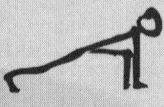

Exhale, stretching one leg back into
Banarasana (high lunge)
Inhale, lengthening from heel to head

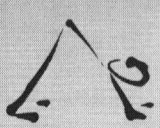

Exhale, pressing back & upward into
Adho Mukha Svanasana (Downward Facing Dog)
Hold while inhaling, exhaling, inhaling again

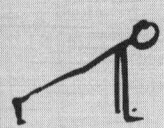

Exhale into
Plank
Inhale in the pose

Illustrations from 108 Yoga Pose Drawings by Charlotte Bradley. Used with permission. Available at yogaflavoredlife.com.

A Yoga Journal

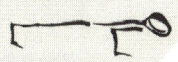

Exhale into
Chaturanga

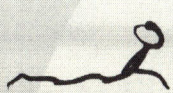

Inhale, bringing chest forward and upward to
Bhujangasana (Cobra, or substitute Sphinx Pose)

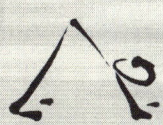

Exhale, pressing back to
Adho Mukha Svanasana (Downward Facing Dog)
Hold while inhaling, exhaling, inhaling again

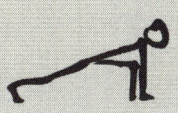

Exhale, stepping foot forward for
Banarasana (high lunge)
Inhale, make sure foot is between hands, not behind

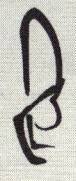

Exhale, stepping other foot forward
Uttanasana (Forward Fold)

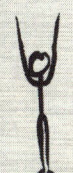

Inhale, stretching arms up
Utthita Tadasana

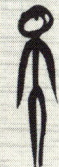

Exhale, lowering arms
Tadasana

Inhale, sweeping arms overhead, and begin again, stepping back into lunge with the opposite foot on the second repetition.

Breathing Techniques

The breath is a bridge between our inner and outer worlds.

We all breathe the same atmosphere, like tugging at different corners of a blanket, so breath connects all living things. The breath is also a bridge between the body's automatic processes (heartbeat, digestion) and the ones we consciously control (walking, talking). It is the easiest of the automatic processes to bring under our deliberate control and then release again.

Yogis call breathwork *Pranayama*. *Prana* is the energy force that sustains life in the body. It flows through channels within and around the body, similar to Chi in acupuncture. The flow of prana is connected to the breath. Through breathing techniques, we can deliberately direct the flow of prana, to energize or calm the nervous system.

Some schools of yoga, such as Iyengar, consider pranayama a very advanced yoga technique and don't teach it until the yogi has full mastery of asana practice. Other styles of yoga incorporate breathwork from the very first class.

The simplest breathing technique is simply to bring awareness to the breath. Inhalations bring energy to the body, and a sense of upward expansion. If you are feeling tired or depressed, try some long, full inhalations with a slight retention at the top. Exhalations bring relaxation, and a downward-pulling energy. When you are feeling agitated or anxious, focus on creating slow, complete exhalations with a slight retention at the bottom.

The breath is a bridge between body and spirit.

Here are three very useful breathing techniques.

Alternate Nostril Breath

For centuries, Yogis have believed that alternate nostril breathing brought balance to the nervous system. Western science caught up in 1994, when experiments proved that breathing through one nostril at a time impacted brain hemisphere activity.

Alternate Nostril Breath (*Nadi Shodhan Pranayama*) brings a sense of peace, often tinged with joy. It is helpful before relaxation or meditation to center the mind, or to free the spirit from stress and agitation.

How to do Alternate Nostril Breathing *(reverse if you are left-handed)*

- Find a comfortable seated position. Press your right nostril closed with your thumb and exhale slowly through the left nostril.

- Inhale through the left nostril (always the same one you just exhaled through), then use your ring finger to gently press the left nostril closed (both nostrils will be closed). Retain the breath comfortably (briefly!). Then lift your thumb away from the right nostril and exhale slowly on the right.

- At the bottom of the exhalation, inhale again through *the same side you've just exhaled through*. Close both nostrils, pause comfortably, then release the left nostril and exhale.

- Continue taking long, smooth, easy breaths through alternate nostrils until you have completed nine rounds of breath (or stop any time you begin to feel uncomfortable). Lower your hand to your lap and enjoy the peaceful feeling for a moment before you begin meditation or continue with your day.

Breath of Joy

Breath of Joy combines movement with breath to build a pleasant sense of energy. It will lift your spirits, countering depression and fatigue. Breath of Joy is a wonderful way to begin a yoga practice, or can be placed at the end of a practice meant to build energy. The breath is made up of a three-part nasal inhalation, with sweeping arm movements, and a noisy exhalation through the mouth as your body folds forward.

How to do Breath of Joy

- Stand with feet hip-width or slightly wider, knees soft. Stay very loose and relaxed, moving like a rag doll.

- Your first inhalation should fill your lungs to about 1/3 of their capacity. Inhale through your nose, creating a strong sniffing sound. As you inhale, swing your relaxed arms forward, parallel to each other at shoulder level or let them cross in front of your chest.

- Without exhaling, take a second sniff of air to fill your lungs to 2/3 capacity, let your arms drop slightly and sweep them out the sides at shoulder level (the arms will make an arc shape as they sweep down and out).

- With your third sniff, complete the inhalation as you sweep your arms forward again, bringing them parallel and floating them overhead, fingertips toward the ceiling.

- Exhale through your mouth with a HHHAAAAA sound. (Some yogis like to use a strong sigh, while others prefer a sharp HA!) As you exhale, bend your knees and let your body fall forward, arms sweeping to your sides and behind you like a skier.

- Let your body rebound back up to standing as you immediately begin the next round of breath.

- Continue for nine rounds of breath, or stop if you begin to feel unpleasantly dizzy or lightheaded.

- Spend a moment in mountain pose, eyes closed, and feel the energy coursing through you.

Breath of Fire

Breath of Fire oxygenates and energizes the entire body and stokes the *Agni* (digestive fire). It also stimulates the solar plexus chakra, so it brings a stronger, more powerful feeling of energy than Breath of Joy. Breath of Fire is used regularly in Kundalini yoga to cleanse the body and spirit.

How to do Breath of Fire

- This should be a relaxed, rhythmic breath that could be maintained for a long time. Advanced practitioners aim for 11 minutes per day! Don't be forceful or rough with the breath.

- Sit straight and tall. Begin breathing through your nose, lightly and shallowly. Let your belly expand when you inhale and your navel move back toward your spine when you exhale.

- The breath is light, rapid, and shallow, with air moving in and out of the top half of your lungs. This technique is sometimes called 'bellows breath' because the diaphragm pumps the air in and out like a bellows.

- The inhalation and exhalation should be of equal duration, force and volume. Make sure not to focus on the exhalation, but keep the breath even, balanced and rhythmic.

- Your diaphragm should be relaxed and the stomach muscles do not contract forcefully (although you can lightly pull your navel toward your spine as you exhale if it helps). The diaphragm should move effortlessly.

- Imagine focusing the breath at the tip of the nose to keep Breath of Fire light and shallow.

- Breath of Fire makes sound. The inhalation sounds like a sniff, the exhalation makes a little blowing sound. Some people think the breath sounds like a steam engine, building power.

- The speed and force of the breath can increase as you become more experienced. Start out at a comfortable pace and work up to 2-3 breaths per second or more.

- Practice for just a minute or two at first.

Chakras

Chakra translates as 'wheel' in Sanskrit. The chakras represent energy centers in the body and are imagined as colored wheels.

Each chakra relates to an endocrine gland and to a group of nerves called a 'plexus.' Think of the chakras as a detailed map of the mind-body connection.

Emotions begin with thoughts and manifest in the chakras. Certain kinds of emotion tend to manifest in specific chakras. Nervousness leads to butterflies in the stomach, sadness or loss to heaviness in the chest, holding back communication gives a lump in the throat.

When tensions continue over time, or at intense levels, physical symptoms can manifest. Chronic anger can lead to heart attacks, or a lifetime of fear might generate an ulcer. These are examples of emotion manifesting around the associated chakra.

Heal your chakras through meditation, breathwork, yoga postures (see pages 16-27) and sound. Deepak Chopra's *Chakra Balancing: Body, Mind, and Soul* CD set has guided meditations for chakra work.

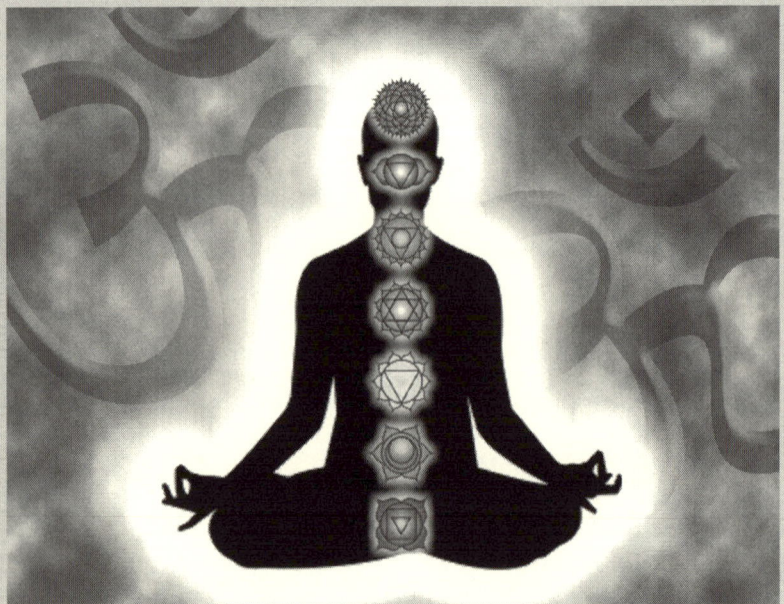

Seated Figure By Bryan Helfrich, via Wikimedia Commons
Chakra symbols by Morgan Phoenix, via Wikimedia Commons

Muladhara (root chakra)

Location: Base of spine, pelvic floor, often visualized with roots through legs. Represents: Security, physical safety. Color: Red. Supported by: Standing poses, grounding meditations.

Svadhisthana (sacral chakra)

Location: Lower belly, in front of the sacrum, below the navel. Represents: Connection to others, sexual feelings, romantic love. Color: Orange. Supported by: Flowing movement, surrendering to gravity in resting poses.

Manipura (solar plexus/power chakra)

Location: Between navel and ribcage. Represents: Willpower, personal strength, self-esteem. Color: Yellow. Supported by: Core work, Breath of Fire, and meditations.

Anahata (heart chakra)

Location: Center of chest. Represents: Compassion, spiritual love. Color: Green. Supported by: Music, meditation, backbending poses.

Vissuddha (throat chakra)

Location: Base of throat, extends through arms. Represents: Communication, creativity. Color: Sky blue. Supported by: Neck stretches, singing, chanting, creating sound.

Ajna (third eye chakra)

Location: Between the eyebrows, an inward-looking eye. Represents: Self-awareness, sixth-sense perception. Color: Indigo. Supported by: Meditation, chanting Ohm, inversions, breathwork.

Sahasrara (crown chakra)

Location: Top of head, space above the crown of the head. Represents: Spirituality, connection to energy and to Divine. Color: Violet, white. Supported by: Meditation, breathwork.

Koshas

If your essential being is a light source, the Koshas are like a series of colored shades that change its appearance (but not its essence). In meditation, we move inward through the koshas to find the source. Note that the koshas are named 'maya' which means appearance, or illusion.

Physical: Annamaya Kosha (Food sheath): In meditation, we become aware of the sensations of the body, explore them, and then go inward toward the other koshas.

Energy: Pranamaya Kosha (Energy Sheath): As the body and mind become quiet, your awareness moves to the subtle movements of energy through the body. Learn to sense and regulate this energy, then go inward.

Mental: Manamaya Kosha (Mind Sheath): Don't underestimate the challenge of learning to keep the mind still as it flits between past and future. The mind is full of doubts and illusions that cloud deeper wisdom.

Wisdom: Vijnanamaya Kosha (Wisdom Sheath): Wisdom is the level of ego consciousness, self-awareness. Wisdom lies beneath the processing of the mind. The Wisdom Sheath allows us to search within for higher levels of consciousness.

Bliss: Anandamaya Kosha (Bliss Sheath): Anandamaya is joy and love that is beyond the mind, independent of any thought or circumstantial happiness. It is simply being, resting in bliss. In deep meditation, this too is released, in order to experience the True Self.

Atman: Self (no Maya, no Sheath): Atman is the Self, the eternal center of consciousness, which was never born and never dies. Your true essence. In our metaphor it is the true light that illuminates all the shades.

What is Ohm?

Imagine that all the energy in the universe is powered by a spiritual generator. Ohm is the hum of that engine.

Ohm is the sound of divine consciousness. It is the seed sound of the universe, of everything that is, has been or will ever be. Ohm is also that which transcends past, present and future. It is the sound that yogis observe when meditation takes them into complete stillness.

Legend says that Ohm was discovered by early yogis when they learned that they were all hearing this sound in their deepest meditative states. Yoga students chant the sound to achieve the same transcendence.

When chanting, think of Ohm as a sound that blends three syllables, A, O, and Mm. The A sound begins deep within the body, and as you transition to the O sound you will feel the vibrations traveling upward. When you finish with the long humming Mm sound, the vibrations move upward into the Third Eye chakra or even the crown chakra area. There is also a hidden fourth sound: the silence that follows Mm.

The *Mandukya Upanishad*, written in 800-500 BC, offers a fascinating breakdown of the Ohm symbol (pictured above). The lower curve (bottom half of the 3) represents our waking, everyday state of consciousness. The top of the 3 denotes dreamless sleep, or meditation. The curly bit between the two represents the state of dreaming, or the mind focused inward. The fourth state, pictured as separate and above the others, is the perfect state of peace: *Samadhi*, or union with the Divine.

This trinity of consciousnesses, with a divine unity that rises above them, parallels the idea of past, present, future and the Divine, which transcends time. It also reflects the three syllables and the silence that follows them.

About Meditation

Some people like to relax with visualizations. They might imagine lying on the beach in the warm sun, or floating lazily down a river. This kind of imaginary escape can help people learn to relax, and even lower their blood pressure. But it is not yoga; in fact, it is the opposite of yoga.

Yoga requires being fully present in your body and in the moment. Meditation, according to Shane-Christopher Perkins of Yandara Yoga Institute, is simple: *Be present. Let go. Over and over.*

In practice, those simple instructions are impossibly difficult to master. That's why we learn a variety of techniques for staying present and for letting go.

Learn to manage your mind

When you begin to meditate, thoughts will intrude. You will be called upon to brush them aside, again and again, without getting frustrated with yourself. Think of your brain as a toddler, resisting naptime. You just have to keep patiently putting it back down until it learns to rest quietly. In the process, you'll learn what kind of chatter arises in your mind. Usually, your thoughts will fall into four categories: reflections on the past, either positive (nostalgia) or negative (guilt, anger) and thoughts about the future, positive (planning, anticipation) or negative (worry).

At some point, as you observe those thoughts and control them by brushing them aside or releasing them with an exhalation, you will also be learning to take control of your mind, and with it your emotions. This is a skill you can use outside of meditation to release negativity and choose joy. Are you inventing awful futures for yourself and putting yourself through pain as if they were real (worrying?). Recognize it, brush it aside, and find something happy to think about! The present moment is nearly always just fine. Stay in it.

Connect with your spirit

Consider that your mind, body and spirit exist separately from one another. But you go through life aware only of your body and your mind and *rarely experience your spirit*. Even people who absolutely believe in 'spirit' as something separate from 'mind' will confuse their spirit with their thoughts.

Your thoughts are not your 'self.' At some point in your attempts to meditate, you have to wonder "Who is this internal observer who can watch and control my thoughts?" It's a fascinating question.

Modern life gives us a constant stream of TV, video games, books, music and other people (in person or on the phone) to distract us from our thoughts. When you sit down to meditate, you will miss those distractions and find your mind alternately boring and a wild mess of constant chatter. It will take a long time to learn to quiet that chatter. At first, finding peace between your thoughts is like finding the dry spaces between raindrops in a storm. Be patient. It will get easier.

If you learn to quiet your mind and body, *you can see what else is present in you*. Just as experiencing your body is different from the way you listen to your mind, your experience of spirit will be very different from what you are used to. It may feel murky at first, a dim perception. But just as turning off the TV lets you turn your attention to your own thoughts, turning off the distraction of the mind lets you turn your attention to your spirit.

Not interested in your spirit? Meditation can still help you discover yourself and learn to control worry, guilt and fear.

Remain present, keep coming back to your body, and keep letting go. The next few pages offer some techniques to help you.

Guided Meditations

Suggestion for using these meditations:

- Read *About Meditation* on pages 164–165.

- Focus on one meditation in depth (perhaps daily for a week) before working with another.

- Read the instructions each time. You will understand them a little more deeply, and remember more, with repetition.

- If you're an auditory person, you might record yourself speaking the instructions. Read slowly, and leave 30 second to 1-minute silences between paragraphs.

- If you have a group to work with, take turns leading the meditation, then share your experiences.

- Use music if you find it relaxing, but not if it distracts you.

- Be comfortable. You cannot meditate if your lower back is throbbing or your body is screaming for release. If long-term floor-sitting isn't for you, sit upright in a chair, or cross-legged on a cushion with a wall to support your back. It's possibly to meditate lying down, but falling asleep is a risk.

- Be warm. As you become more relaxed, your extremities will get cold. Pull on warm socks or wrap a meditation shawl around yourself.

- Having a specific location, cushion, shawl, music, or scent that triggers meditation for you will help speed the process.

- Start with just a few minutes at a time. Meditation should feel like a treat, not a torture. You will enjoy sitting for longer periods as your skills develop.

Savasana (Relaxation) Meditation

Perfect for beginners, during Savasana, or as a way to feel centered before a more complex meditation. This meditation will teach you how to relax, how to let go, and how to use your body as an 'anchor' to quiet your mind. Recline on the floor, with cushions under your thighs or knees and a rolled towel under your neck. Cover up with a blanket.

Close your eyes. Turn your attention inward.

Take your awareness to the soles of your feet. Imagine the soles of your feet softening, toes relaxing. Soften the tops of your feet. Relax your ankles and lower legs. Let go of any holding around the knees and thighs. Relax all the way from the hip joints to the toes. Feel the weight of your hips and legs as you surrender your lower body to gravity.

Allow your belly and chest to rise and fall together gently with your breath. Soften your side ribs and side waist, allow your front body to rest against your back body as your back body softens against the floor. Imagine warmth and relaxation radiating through your lower back, midback, and across your shoulder blades. Give the weight of both shoulders to the earth. Allow this sense of relaxation to flow into your upper arms, forearms, wrists and hands. Soften your fingers, backs of your hands and palms.

Feel your neck soften and lengthen as you surrender the weight of your head to gravity. Release your jaw, allowing teeth to separate behind closed lips. Relax your tongue. See if you can feel or imagine the sensation of relaxing the roof of your mouth. Soften the back of your throat.

Smooth your cheeks, eyelids, and forehead. Let go of tiny muscles under your scalp and around your ears. Find your inner ears and soften them. Behind closed eyelids, lower your gaze and let your awareness drop from your brain into your heart center or belly.

Focus on your exhalations. Create long, slow, gentle exhalations. Feel the weight of your back body against the floor. When you mind begins to wander, come back to the exhalations. Let yourself sink more deeply into gravity and into relaxation with each exhalation.

Scan your body and release tension wherever you find it — even if you need to patiently let go of the same spot over and over.

Become aware of the pause at the bottom of each exhalation: that moment when you're no longer exhaling, and you're not holding the breath, but it's not necessary yet to inhale. See if you can use that pause to let yourself sink more deeply within.

Gradually shift your awareness to your inhalations. Imagine bringing life force and energy into the lungs with each inhalation. As you exhale, imagine spreading that energy out to every cell of the body, every finger and toe.

As you take your awareness out to the fingers and toes, start making small movements there, circling the wrists and ankles. If you like, you can reach your arms overhead and stretch. Then roll onto your right side and rest there for a moment.

When you're ready, use your hands and arms to help you come up to a seated position. Keep your head and neck relaxed. Open your eyes, letting light in without sending energy out.

Energy Meditation

For some people, this meditation is simply a visualization that keeps their focus firmly in the physical body and quiets the mind. For scientific types, it's an interesting exploration of respiration at the cellular level. For others, energy awareness is a very real and intense experience. Your experience is perfect, exactly as it is.

Find a comfortable seat and turn your attention inward, eyes closed. Focus on your breath until your mind begins to settle and your body is relaxed.

Gradually bring your awareness to the crown of your head. Imagine that you can feel the subtle movements of air across your scalp. Imagine being able to perceive the tingle of energy in the room through your crown. As you inhale, imagine pulling energy into your body through the top of your head. Soften your throat and the roof of your mouth, and inhale a beam of light and energy that passes through the crown of your head, drawing it down into your heart center. With each inhalation, let that beam of golden light and energy become brighter and more powerful, creating a reservoir of energy around your heart center. Drink energy through the top of your head as if you are sipping light through a straw.

When the visualization is strong and the top of your head feels engaged with the energy in the room, begin using your exhalations to push the light downward. Light up your belly and hips, your legs. Press the energy all the way down and out through the soles of your feet. You can move energy through your arms as well, letting it exit through your palms.

Imagine lighting up all the darkness within. Imagine being so filled with light that your skin gives off a glow. Let the light and energy within you expand beyond the boundaries of your physical body.

Let the meditation take you where it will from there.

Note: Some students have a better experience reclining in Savasana and 'drinking' energy in reverse, bringing it in through the soles of their feet and up to their heart center on the inhalations, then flowing it out through the palms of the hands and crown with each exhalation. This can be a very grounding practice, and is sometimes easier for beginners.

If you have a partner, experiment with lying down with the soles of your feet or the crowns of your heads very close together. See if you can feel energy flowing between you.

Knowledge

Koshas: A Falling Inward Meditation

Reread the information about Koshas on page 172. Don't expect to pass through all the koshas on your first try, or your hundredth try. It will happen when it happens.

Sit comfortably, eyes closed, and bring your awareness to your body. Ground yourself in the feeling of your weight in your hips and legs. When you feel relaxed and centered, let your awareness move to your Energy Sheath. Rather than trying to direct your energy, simply follow it with your attention. What happens to the energy flowing through and around you when you inhale? What happens when you exhale?

After observing your energy for a while, shift your awareness to your Mental Sheath. What sort of chatter is filling up your mind and trying to distract you? Rather than trying to stop your mental chatter, let it become a background noise that you ignore, turning your attention elsewhere.

Allow yourself to become aware of that part of you that is observing and directing your thoughts. Spend a little time pondering the relationship between this inner observer and the thoughts s/he directs. Then let go of this level of thought as well. Turn tour attention inward as if you are waiting for your eyes to adjust to darkness, certain you will become aware of something else soon. Keep relaxing your body and remaining present, without letting the chatter in your mind capture your attention, as you look within. Become aware of your fear of leaving your thoughts behind, and imagine that fear as a thin barrier within you that prevents you from going deeper. Exhale and imagine gently pressing through that barrier and sinking deeper within yourself. If you find yourself in a sea of pure bliss, stay there for a while. Let the bliss wash over you and flow through you until you are ready to go deeper. Then imagine your resistance to letting go of the bliss as another thin membrane within you. Exhale and let yourself sink through that barrier to see what else is present.

Lovingkindness Meditation

This is a variation on a traditional Buddhist meditation that cultivates internal joy. Kindle feelings of love and warmth, then expand and extend those feelings. See if you can keep one toe in that pool of lovingkindness throughout your day.

Sit comfortably with eyes closed. Begin by thinking of something innocent, something you can easily extend loving feelings toward without expecting anything in return. Perhaps a warm puppy, wiggling with joy. Or maybe a sleeping infant, or a toddling kitten. Find the experience of love and warmth in your heart and explore it. Where in your body do you experience love? What does it feel like? Does this feeling have a shape, a size, a color? Does it move upward, downward, expand, or contract?

Let go of the image but keep the feeling. Allow the loving feelings to wash over you as you say to yourself "May I be peaceful, happy and safe."

Now think of someone you are grateful to, someone you feel warm towards, and direct the loving feeling toward them. Say to yourself, "May s/he be peaceful, happy and safe."

Inhale and imagine your heart center expanding, like a bubble, large enough to enfold your family, or the people who share your house, building, or street. Exhale and let your love wash over them. "May they be peaceful, happy and safe." Continue expanding your heart center to include your neighborhood, your city, your state, your country.

Think of someone you don't like, or who is giving you a hard time. It is very empowering to send love to the people who have hurt or upset you. You don't have to forgive them, just wish them well. "May they be peaceful, happy, and safe."

Finally, open your heart to the world, the universe. "May all beings everywhere be happy." Throughout the day, see if you can turn your attention inward for a moment to recover this feeling of lovingkindness.

Dissipating Negative Emotions

This is more of a technique than a meditation, but it is so valuable I thought it was important to share it with you. As you build awareness of your mind, body and spirit, you will be able to use your skills to manage your most devastating emotions. You can 'practice' this technique by remembering a difficult time, dwelling on it until emotion rises within you. If you are in great emotional pain, it can be helpful to have a friend sit with you and ask these questions.

Remember, emotions are physical manifestations of thought.

While experiencing a strong negative emotion, close your eyes and turn your attention inward. Where do you feel this emotion? Is it in your head, throat, chest, belly, pelvis? *(Note that emotions tend to manifest around the chakras. No one feels fear in their wrists.)*

What does it look and feel like? Can you describe it? Move your awareness away from your thoughts, by focusing on the sensation in your body completely. How large is it? Does it have a shape? A color? Is it warm, or cold, or does it have no temperature? Does it have movement? Upward, downward, contracting, expanding, spinning?

Let go of the story in your mind, the reason for the feeling, and just become curious about the feeling itself.

Can you bring some breath around it? Some space? Can your breath soften the edges of the sensation? Can you gradually vaporize its edges and make it smaller?

Do you want it to go away, or do you find yourself clinging to it?

Use long, slow breaths to calm yourself and to dissipate the emotion. Release a little more of it with each exhalation, until it shrinks away to nothing and vanishes in a final wisp of steam.

Sit a little while longer, enjoying your breath and using your favorite meditation techniques to fill yourself with peace and light.

About the Author

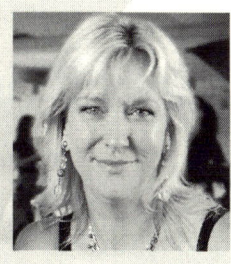

Lauren "Zehara" Haas is a third-generation yogini. She grew up unaware that other families didn't have stretching time on the floor or talk about meditation.

When changes in the economy ended her career as a local magazine publisher, Lauren decided it was time to stop trying to make things happen and settle into allowing a new career to unfold. Much to her surprise, her passion for Middle Eastern dance began to take over her life. Soon she was making a full-time living as a bellydance performer and teacher. Utimately Lauren owned two world dance/yoga studios, plus taught at an international conference and on a cruise ship in the Indian Ocean.

Lauren went to Yandara Yoga Institute in Baja, Mexico in 2004 to earn a yoga teaching certification. A month of living in the desert, studying yoga full-time with the Yandara teachers, gave her much more than she bargained for, opening her spirit as well as her mind and body.

After over a decade as a dance and yoga instructor, Lauren traded her studios and performance career for a nomadic life as a freelance writer. Lauren writes extensively for CBS and Time Warner. This is her second book.

Also by Lauren "Zehara" Haas

- A Belly Dance Journal
- Stage Presence With Lauren Zehara (a DVD for bellydancers)

Coming Soon!

- **Bliss: Guided Meditations**, an audio CD

Printed in Great Britain
by Amazon.co.uk, Ltd.,
Marston Gate.